Garry Trainer

www.garrytrainer.com

With more than twenty years of clinical experience as an osteopath, acupuncturist and masseur, Garry Trainer says he has to give out the same advice to patients time and time again.

Originally from New Zealand, Garry was a budding sportsman until a serious back injury struck at the age of seventeen. After three months in hospital and eighteen months of drugs and conventional medical treatment, Garry was devastated. Gone were the days of surfing and playing rugby and he was also unable to continue his career as a nurse because lifting anyone was impossible.

Garry came to England in 1979 and trained as an acupuncturist at the London School of Chinese Medicine and then as an osteopath at the Andrew Stills College. Today, he lives part time in London and Marlow, running successful practices in Harley Street and Primrose Hill.

He has been featured in many newspapers and magazines and has made numerous appearances on television and radio. Often known as the celebrity back doctor, Garry has treated Sir Paul McCartney, Gwyneth Paltrow, Kate Winslet, Emma Thompson, Depeche Mode, Sam Neill, Rupert Everett, George Michael, Dire Straits, Eric Clapton, Coldplay, Lou Reed, Sir Anthony Sher, Brad Pitt, Robbie Williams, the Eagles, Sir Ian Holm, Jahangar Khan and Ed Moses and has also been retained by the Royal Shakespeare Company.

Tania Alexander

Tania Alexander is a freelance health journalist and consumer expert, who has been writing for national newspapers for nearly twenty years. She met Garry when she interviewed him about back pain for *Sunday Times Style* and was subsequently his co-author for *The No-Nonsense Guide to a Healthy Back*. She writes regularly in the 'Good Health' section of the *Daily Mail* and has been one of their health writers for many years.

Tania brings her research skills to this book, providing the most up-to-date and accurate information on back pain, products and treatment methods. She is also a trained YMCA fitness instructor and author of six books. She lives in London with her husband and three children.

THE ULTIMATE GUIDE TO HEALING
AND PREVENTING BACK PAIN

BackChat

GARRY TRAINER AND TANIA ALEXANDER

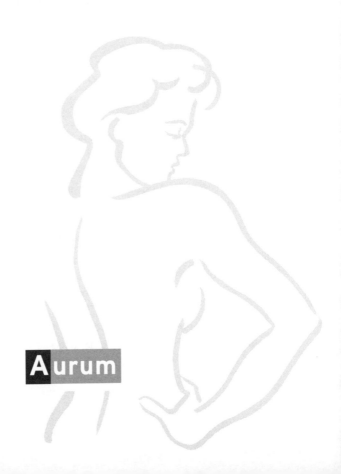

Aurum

First published in Great Britain
2007 by Aurum Press Limited
25 Bedford Avenue
London WC1B 3AT

A catalogue record for this book is available from the British Library.

ISBN-10: 1 84513 208 4
ISBN-13: 978 1 84513 208 8

10 9 8 7 6 5 4 3 2 1
2011 2010 2009 2008 2007

Although every effort has been made to ensure that the contents of this book are accurate, it must not be treated as a substitute for qualified medical advice. Always consult a qualified medical practitioner. Neither the authors nor the publisher can be held responsible for any loss or claim arising out of the use or misuse of the suggestions made or the failure to take medical advice.

Text design by Rich Carr
Illustrations by Connie Jude
Photography by Philip Wilkins
Printed and bound in Great Britain by MPG Books, Bodmin

This book is printed on paper certified by the Forest Stewardship Council as coming from a forest that is well managed according to strict environmental, social and economic standards.

Dedications

Garry Trainer
To my little mini me, Max

Tania Alexander
To Alex, Anoushka and Joshua

Contents

Foreword
Dr Hilary Jones

There are three good reasons why I can recommend this excellent book. Firstly, as a GP I know just how common backache is amongst the general population as well as how socially inconvenient and physically disabling it can be. No two people's back pain is the same, yet all too often patients are categorized under the umbrella title and treated along identical lines. Orthodox medicine is not good at sorting out a precise diagnosis and is even worse at coming up with a practical and logical treatment plan with a view to getting the patient pain-free and mobilized so that they can enjoy their normal lifestyle. Consequently frustration and depression caused by chronic pain is widespread.

Secondly, my insight into the modern management of back pain has been more sharply focussed by suffering from it from time to time myself. Competitive rowing and regular squash are probably not conducive to a normal healthy ramrod spine, and over the years I have responded to my own back pain in a variety of ways. Trying to ignore it, giving up exercise, seeing ineffective doctors, acupuncture, lumbar supports and massage, medication, changes of mattress, anti-gravity devices, physiotherapy, several epidurals and osteopathy all feature, which brings me on to my third point, Garry Trainer.

I was first introduced to Garry at GMTV and formed an instant rapport with a man who was obviously extremely knowledgeable and who enjoyed an awesome reputation amongst all of his clients, both of the ordinary and celebrity kind. The second time I met him, I did what many people do to me, and asked him if whilst he was there he could carry out a quick manipulation on my very painful neck. He duly complied, and within five minutes I walked away pain free with a full range of neck movement. If that isn't medical magic, I don't know what is.

Since then, we have shared many patients and I'm delighted to introduce this superb and very clear and concise book which is a must for anyone wanting to know more about back pain and self-manage it. I recommend it to everyone.

Introduction
by Garry Trainer

Back pain is a part of modern life. Almost eighty per cent of people will experience back pain at some time during their lives. When back pain strikes, it can feel that your whole life is tipped upside down. All the little things you took for granted suddenly become an obstacle. Getting dressed, sitting comfortably on the sofa, going for a walk or even getting out of bed can suddenly become a huge hurdle. You may even feel that life will never be the same again!

I might be sitting on the other side of the fence now but I've been there in terms of experiencing severe back pain. I come from New Zealand and when I was seventeen I sustained a terrible rugby injury, which badly damaged my back. It was caused by a tackle with two big burly props, in which I found myself caught in the middle while they both went in different directions. I was taken straight to hospital and admitted to the spinal unit where I had to stay for three months. It was such a depressing time: everyone had a wheelchair next to their bed and there were periods when there was no feeling in my legs at all. I really thought I might never lead a normal life again.

But I did, and through the healing process I learnt an awful lot, which I hope to impart to you in this book. There are so many ways to tackle back pain. Hopefully this book will give you the power and confidence to do so.

So what makes this book different from other back books? It is not a medical textbook. Instead of bombarding you with too much scientific detail, which frankly I don't believe anyone needs, Tania and I concentrated on the core information about how this amazing structure – your back – works and the best ways to protect it. We have also included lots of case histories so that you can see that you are not alone and can pick up some advice from people with similar problems. I've commented on each one and given treatment and lifestyle tips.

Whether or not you are currently having treatment for a back problem, you should find this book useful. In fact, I believe that everyone should read this book at least once! Even if you are one of the lucky ones who has never suffered from back pain, you will find plenty of information in the book to keep your spine healthy. It should also make useful reading for anyone living with someone with back pain – providing a chance to really identify with what the other person is going through. Back pain is not life-threatening but it certainly can threaten the quality of your life. Of course, no book is a substitute for going to see a doctor or back specialist, so if you still feel worried or confused you should always consult a professional.

The spine is the backbone of your health. Look after it and it will look after you.

You're not alone

- Back pain has a huge impact on industry and society – by reading through our case histories, you will see what a cross section of people are struck by it.

- It is estimated that up to four out of five people will experience back pain lasting more than a day at some time during their lives.

- Back pain is one of the world's leading causes of disability, affecting 1.1 million people in the UK – more than any other condition.

- Almost half the adult population in the UK report low-grade back pain, lasting for at least twenty-four hours, at some point in the year.

- Nearly 120 million working days are lost every year in the UK because of back pain, at a cost of £6 billion each year.

- Back pain is also very prevalent in children: recent research by the charity BackCare found that fifty per cent of schoolchildren suffer from back pain.

- Up to ten per cent of children in every class suffer chronic or recurrent back pain that is bad enough to compromise their involvement in sporting activities, school attendance, self-esteem, relationships and future quality of life.

- Back pain is the second most common cause of long-term sick leave for the population in general and the most common for people in manual occupations.

CHAPTER 1

The back demystified

There is something very mystical about the back, and in particular the spine, which is the central supporting system of your body. The spine supplies nerves to every organ and muscle in the body and is therefore a very important structure and one well worth looking after. When your back is working properly, you probably never think about it. But when something goes wrong, the whole of your being can be affected.

Your back is actually much stronger than you might think. Everyone has an excellent self-healing mechanism, which is often all that is needed in order to get through a bout of back pain. In most cases there is really no need for treatment. Time is often the greatest healer and, given time, the back will generally do a good job in healing itself. (Once upon a time, before there were skilled medical practitioners, time was all you had to fix things.)

One of the aims of this book is to demystify the back and to take the fear out of your pain. It really is not so complicated to understand. We have deliberately not gone into too many medical details but have concentrated on providing concise information about how the back works and what you can do to keep it healthy and mobile, especially as some of you may be in so much pain that even sitting reading this book may be agonizing.

So let's start by cutting it down to basics.

HOW DOES THE BACK WORK?

Your back is designed to move in six directions: forwards, backwards, laterally left and right and rotationally clockwise and anti-clockwise. These movements can also be combined.

At the core of your back is your spine, which is more substantial than many people imagine – it's actually deep-set and takes up about half of the body's diameter. The spinal column is made up of a graceful column of thirty-three bones called vertebrae, plus the sacrum and coccyx at the base. The spine curves in a smooth 'S'-shape. The back of it comprises the individual spines of vertebrae, which you can feel through the skin. Each vertebra moves with the vertebrae above and below it. When these normally mobile joints get stuck, problems arise.

The spine is strengthened by ligaments, which run down the length of it, and is supported by muscles, which attach to the vertebrae through tendons. In between each vertebra is a disc, which acts as a shock absorber, and nerve roots, which feed nerve supply to the whole body.

The spine also acts as casing to protect the vital and fragile spinal cord, part of the central nervous system, which runs down the inside of the spinal column from the base of the brain.

WHAT CAUSES BACK PAIN?

There are many structures in the back that can cause pain and each one of these has a unique pattern of symptoms. For example, the most likely structure in the back to cause pins and needles and numbness is a nerve.

Musculoskeletal pain

Musculoskeletal (also known as 'mechanical') pain is the most common type of back pain. When it first comes on, this sort of pain can be very acute but from then on it's a more low-grade pain that some people describe as an ache or niggling pain that's mainly felt in the muscle. If you have injured a back muscle it will initially hurt when you move it. As the healing process continues, however, movement can actually bring some pain relief to the area as it increases circulation. The underlying principle of all physical therapy is to improve blood supply to the affected area. This can be done in a variety of ways, the most common being massage, heat lamps and ultrasound. At home you can take a hot bath or shower or use a special heat patch or lamp. A simple heat-rub product can be effective and some gentle stretching after the first few days is also a good idea.

Acupuncture (see pages 62–3) achieves the same result by bringing blood flow to the area of incision. Whenever something foreign is embedded in the skin (this could be a splinter, thorn or sterile needle), the body reacts by sending an increased blood supply to the area to fight off potential infection. Acupuncture uses the same mechanism but for a different purpose.

Without any treatment most musculoskeletal problems show signs of improvement after a few days and can then completely disappear within seven to ten days. The role of treatment is simply to speed up this self-healing process.

Nerve pain

The telltale sign that a nerve is involved is numbness, pins and needles or pain in another area of the body that is connected by that nerve. (This is known as 'referred pain'.) In severe cases of nerve compression you may feel more pain down the extremity of the nerve (for example in the lower leg) than in the back itself. You may also lose reflexes and strength in the muscles fed by this nerve.

Any movement or exercise will aggravate this type of back pain, so avoid it. Ice treatments work best: an ice pack at the end of the day can be particularly beneficial. Surrounding muscles may have gone into spasm as a way of protecting you from further damage. Nerves are much more sensitive than muscles, so if pain persists it would be worthwhile seeing a specialist. Once the pressure is released from the nerve, the pain should be alleviated, but it can take several weeks for the inflammation to settle down.

Disc pain

The discs are the shock absorbers between the vertebrae. A disc is fairly robust as its gel-like nucleus allows it to change shape according to the pressure put upon it.

If a disc is overloaded by a sudden change of position, lifting a heavy weight or just carrying excess body weight, however, it can tear and rupture, causing extreme pain. The most common way to injure a disc is through a twisting action or by lifting a heavy object awkwardly. Just bending forwards can injure a disc. If the injury is severe, the disc fluid will start to seep out and may cause compression of the spinal cord, the ligaments or the nerve roots – all extremely painful. Discs degenerate with age, which is why middle-aged people are so susceptible to problems with them.

Disc problems are best treated with lots of rest and passive treatments such as acupuncture for pain relief. It is important, though, to make sure you keep mobile in order to maintain circulation to the affected area. If this is too painful to achieve on your own you may need a therapist to help you. If the disc is ruptured and putting pressure on the spinal cord, surgery may be needed. If so, don't panic – less than ten per cent of back injuries actually result in surgery and surgical techniques nowadays are very effective and safe.

CASE HISTORY ❶

Whiplash

Rachel, 37, designer

The problem

Whiplash can throw the neck in an awkward position, thereby trapping a nerve and straining local soft tissue.

The solution

If the accident was not very severe, this may not need treatment and may heal itself with rest, but you can alleviate some of the pain by going to see an osteopath or similar practitioner to release the nerve. Watch out for any lingering or worsening symptoms, such as headaches, blurred vision or dizziness because these may be a sign of something more serious and needs to be investigated by a doctor.

My case was both strange and frightening. I was working for a month in New York when I started getting the most terrible headaches. Every time I lay down, my head would start spinning. I put it down to bad jet lag but it never cleared up. I was too scared and busy to get it seen to while I was away. When I came back to England, I went straight to my GP, who said I needed to have a series of tests including an MRI scan. The worry was that I might have a tumour. Much to my relief, all the tests came back negative yet the problem still continued. It was fine when I was sitting or standing but every time I lay down I felt as though the ceiling was whirring. I had to be very careful getting up or it would set it off more – I would try to hold my head and keep it very still. It used to take ages for me to get up and ready in the morning.

I went back to my GP, who thought it could be a nerve trapped in my neck. She recommended I see Garry, who made the link between a minor car accident I had in New York and the dizziness. All my problems seemed to be coming from my neck and spine as a result of the whiplash. It was such a relief to think we had found the cause and that it wasn't anything more sinister. It took three sessions before the spinning sensation became much less intense. By the fifth session the problem had gone completely.

Garry says: Osteopathy is perfect for releasing a trapped nerve exiting from the spine which may be irritated by a joint that has become locked or stuck. Many people experience an immediate relief once the joint surfaces have been freed. It can take some time, though, for the inflammation to recede from the nerve, which is what happened in Rachel's case and why she needed more than one treatment. The muscles in Rachel's neck had gone into spasm, which is the body's way of protecting itself from further damage by not allowing movement to pass through the area.

It's human nature to always imagine the worst scenario and this is exactly what Rachel was doing. In her panic she had forgotten to look carefully at what had happened in the preceding weeks, which meant she missed the connection between the car accident and the whiplash symptoms that followed. With back pain, you always need to look at what has happened or changed in the last few weeks. Whiplash, for example, can throw the neck forwards, backwards or to the side and can trap a nerve, causing symptoms such as dizziness, headaches or blurred vision.

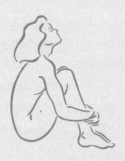

CASE HISTORY ❷

A trapped nerve

Diane, 28, PR director

The problem

A trapped nerve in the neck is commonly caused by poor posture or sleeping in an awkward position.

The solution

As unpleasant as a trapped nerve is, it will sometimes heal on its own depending on how badly the nerve is being irritated. Allow three days to see if it improves before seeking treatment. After it has healed, try to identify the root cause – you may have been sleeping on the wrong type of pillow, for example – and amend your lifestyle accordingly.

I never had any back pain but suddenly found myself with a stiff, painful neck. It was a disaster as I run my own company and have two kids so I don't have a lot of time to take care of myself. I took stacks of painkillers – none of which worked – and then tried to ignore the pain. But after a couple of weeks it was getting worse and I had also lost sensation in my fingers. My GP said she thought I had a trapped nerve and suggested I see an osteopath.

The best thing about going for treatment was finding out exactly what was wrong, as secretly I had been worried sick. The osteopath went through my medical history and then checked my neck and the reflexes in my arms. The loss of sensation in my fingers helped him track the pain, which was apparently travelling down from my neck. He asked lots of questions and finally made a link between the pain and the fact that I had recently invested in some new pillows.

After the first treatment, my neck felt almost instantly better. In about four days it totally healed up and I haven't had any problems since. Next time I would be less stoical and go and see someone sooner.

Garry says: This is a classic case of a trapped nerve, which can usually be treated very successfully with osteopathy. Although in many cases a trapped nerve will eventually heal up on its own, treatment can help accelerate the process and therefore minimize the pain.

Diane was experiencing pins and needles and numbness in the fingers – classic signs that there is neural involvement and that the trapped nerve is quite bad. Although these sensations can be quite scary, they also help make the diagnosis easier as the practitioner will be able to tell exactly which nerve is involved. There are only three nerves passing down the arm: the ulna nerve feeds the small finger and ring finger, the medial nerve feeds the middle finger, and the radial nerve feeds the thumb and forefinger. In Diane's case it was the radial nerve, which exits between the fifth and sixth cervical vertebrae, that was the source of the problem.

I checked her range of movement – there was limited rotation to the left and a sharp pain between the fifth and sixth cervical vertebrae. This was an indication that the vertebrae were stuck to the right so I turned her head to the left and applied a small thrust to release the fixation on the right-hand side where the nerve was being irritated.

As I explained to Diane, pain relief does not address the actual cause. In her case the pain was obviously too severe to be helped by an over-the-counter medication. The pain could be relieved only once pressure was taken off the nerve.

Neck pain can result from very innocent causes, such as sitting in a draught or sleeping on too many pillows. In Diane's case, I discovered that she had changed the pillow she was used to sleeping on and the new one must have been too high.

It is good to sleep on a small firm pillow in order to prevent neck pain (see page 171). My brother will not travel anywhere without his favourite pressure moulding pillow. If you are prone to neck problems, find a pillow that you are comfortable with, stick with it and be prepared to find room for it in your suitcase!

A slipped disc

Jane, 36, marketing manager

The problem
The outer edge of a disc can rupture and the fluid within can seep out, causing extreme pain.

The solution
Time is the best healer in this scenario. A low-grade slipped disc can heal itself in six to eight weeks. Treatment such as traction can help relieve the constant compression of gravity. Rest is imperative, so you may need to take time off work and get someone to help you at home.

I slipped a disc about four years ago. It crept up on me slowly until one morning I was in so much pain I couldn't even get dressed. My husband was away on business but fortunately my mother was staying with us. She helped me into the car and I lay on the back seat all the way to the hospital, screaming. They packed me off with anti-inflammatories, painkillers and muscle relaxants and told me to go to my GP to arrange a scan. The consultant confirmed that I had a slipped disc and that I was unlikely to get better without an operation.

At that point I was in so much pain I couldn't walk for more than a minute. Yet I didn't want to have to undergo surgery. A physiotherapist friend of mine suggested I get a second opinion. The consultant orthopaedic surgeon I saw advised me to avoid an operation at all costs. He said my back would heal itself in time and an operation would involve cutting through muscle, which would weaken my back in the future. He would recommend surgery only if the problem kept occurring. Fortunately I was able to work from home and after a few weeks the pain did slowly start to subside.

Two years later I was five months pregnant and the whole problem flared up again. It wasn't quite as bad as the first time but I didn't want to take painkillers in case they affected the baby. When my daughter was about five months old, it happened for the third time. The pain was so bad I could not even pick her up and I had to feed her lying down. I had to have my mother and aunties to help me.

I went to see a couple of osteopaths but they did not seem to help and gave me conflicting diagnoses. One said it was the slipped disc again, the other that it was my sacroiliac joint. I got to the point where the pain had plateaued but wasn't getting any better. It was only when I finally started getting treated by Garry, who gave me acupuncture and worked ever so gently on the problem, that the pain began to subside. After our second session I was well enough to come off the painkillers. It was such a relief. I was afraid I would never get better. With back problems like this the constant nagging pain really grinds you down. Hopefully my back problems are now over.

Garry says: I always advise patients with disc problems not to immediately jump at the idea of surgery. Time is a great healer and often even a very bad back like Jane's can resolve itself in six to eight weeks. Some discs just swell rather than rupture, which was evidently the case with Jane. Time and conservative management can assist such a disc back to normality.

Jane is very slender so any treatment had to be very soft and gentle. I used a lot of acupuncture on her – when she first came to see me I could hardly lay my hands on her without her screaming in pain. It is very scary to endure the pain of a disc problem without someone in the home to help. If you do live on your own, you will probably need to call on the help of a friend or relative. When you can't pick up your own baby, for example, you can feel useless, which in time can make you feel quite depressed. Patience is the order of the day when it comes to disc problems. It is not something that is going to heal overnight.

Ligament pain

Ligaments act as stabilizers by holding the bones together. They are elastic structures but there is a limit to the amount of stretch that they will take. Regular stretching will help keep your ligaments strong and healthy. Most low-grade back pain is caused by prolonged overstretching of ligaments, which can occur through poor postural habits such as sitting in a slumped position or lying on a sagging mattress. Ligaments normally heal themselves through rest and will become as strong as before as long as they are not overstretched too soon. With age, ligaments will lose their elasticity, which may produce a low-grade ache. Unfortunately, there is nothing that can be done to help this.

Joint pain

The function of a joint is to enable the body to move and be flexible so joints act a bit like hinges in the body, positioned where the bones meet. They are supported by the ligaments. Back pain is often the result of a joint that is stuck; cracking it (see page 58) can provide instant relief. Cracking a joint involves pulling the surfaces apart and promoting the flow of synovial fluid, which relieves the pain.

Arthritis is the most common joint problem. It covers a range of inflammatory and degenerative conditions that cause stiffness, swelling and pain in the joints, particularly in the fingers, hips and knees. Arthritis can occur wherever two joint surfaces rub together and the protective cartilage layer is worn away. In extreme cases, a joint can be replaced with surgery. The best way to relieve pain in the joint is through a combination of heat (increases circulation) and ice (reduces inflammation), both of which desensitize the pain.

There are over 100 different types of arthritis conditions. The best known are osteoarthritis and rheumatoid arthritis, and you will usually need a consultation with an expert such as a rheumatologist to determine which yours is.

Rheumatoid arthritis is an autoimmune disease in which your own immune system attacks healthy tissues, causing inflammation that damages the joints. Classic symptoms include redness of the joints, swelling, tenderness, prolonged morning stiffness and restricted movement. Often genetic, it is three times more common in women than in men and can affect people of all ages. It tends to occur in episodes, which can last for several weeks or months. Medication will be prescribed according to the severity of the condition, with the aim of controlling the symptoms and reducing pain.

Osteoarthritis, also known as 'degenerative' arthritis, is the result of wear and tear and is caused by breakdown of cartilage. It usually affects middle-aged and older people and is twice as common in women than in men. Past injuries and being overweight are both risk factors of osteoarthritis. It is also common in former athletes, gymnasts and dancers due to the extra strain they have put on their joints. Osteoarthritis usually affects the main weight-bearing joints of the body, such as hips, knees and ankles (hands, feet and the spine are also often affected), so high-impact exercise should be avoided and substituted by non-weight-bearing exercise such as swimming. Regular swimming helps maintain mobility of joints and cardiovascular fitness and strengthens the muscles without straining your joints.

Cervical spondylosis is a form of osteoarthritis that affects the joints in the neck resulting in bony spurs and problems with ligaments and discs. Pain in the neck is common and may be a natural consequence of ageing. Like the rest of the body, bones in the neck (cervical spine) progressively degenerate as we grow older. The spinal canal may also narrow (stenosis), compressing the spinal cord and nerves to the arms. The pain that results may range from mild discomfort to severe, crippling dysfunction.

Ankylosing spondylitis is an inflammation and stiffness in the joints, commonly affecting the spine and pelvis. It is four times more common in men than in women and usually starts in late adolescence or early adulthood. In severe cases, new bone grows between the vertebrae in the spine, which eventually fuses them together. It can also distort the spine, resulting in a stooped posture. It is often a genetic disease, something that can be checked by a blood test. If x-rays show any new bone growth, anti-inflammatory drugs may be prescribed in addition to special exercises to help strengthen the back.

Summary

- Your back is an important structure that is worth looking after – if something goes wrong it can affect your whole being.

- The spine is the central supporting system of your body. It is made up of individual bones (vertebrae), which are supported by ligaments and strengthened by muscles, and it protects the spinal cord, which is part of the central nervous system.

- There are many structures in the back that can cause pain and each has a unique pattern of symptoms.

- Everyone has an excellent self-healing mechanism, which is often all that is needed to get through a bout of pain – for many types of back pain, time is the best healer.

CHAPTER 2

What to do when back pain strikes

Before you settle down and read further into this book, there's one thing we'd like to stress: don't give yourself a hard time – you feel bad enough as it is! It's not always your fault that you've got back pain. Many people react to back injury by asking themselves, 'What have I done?' There is often a sense of failure and victimization. Everyone else seems to be moving freely and you just can't.

You probably didn't do anything dramatic at all. It may well be the result of an accumulation of stresses or of simply making the wrong movement at the wrong time. Perhaps you sneezed, coughed or moved awkwardly. The very fact that we move means we have to expect mechanical problems at some time through overuse, misuse or abuse.

Most people will get back pain at some time in their lives. If your back suddenly goes, it can be terrifying not knowing what to do, particularly the first time it happens. But don't panic! By the time you finish reading this book, and in particular this chapter, you should feel greatly reassured. In most cases, the back problem will sort itself out – providing you rest. Follow the advice in this chapter, and after three days you should normally start to feel a lot better again. Believe in your back – it can often heal itself if you give it the right conditions.

Ten common causes

- Doing something you're not used to

- A sedentary lifestyle

- Sitting or standing for prolonged periods

- Sleeping awkwardly

- Lifting something heavy

- Pregnancy

- Coughing or sneezing

- Repetitive movements

- Driving

- Getting older

THE FIRST TWENTY-FOUR HOURS

Suddenly finding yourself in a spasm – doubled up with pain and unable to move – can be one of the scariest things to cope with when you first get back pain. However, it is important to realize that muscle spasm is the body's natural way of protecting itself, by preventing any movement that could go through to the more sensitive underlying structures. It might not feel like it at the time, but you are actually incredibly lucky that this mechanism is in place and working because it is preventing further damage.

The golden rule for this first twenty-four hours is to take it easy. If you've always fancied being a slob for a day, now is your chance! Lie flat on your back, ideally on a firm surface. A bed is fine providing the mattress really is firm and not sagging, otherwise lie on the floor. Make sure you have everything you need to hand so that you can just stay there and rest as much as possible for the first twenty-four hours. It is also important to ensure some movement to aid circulation, even if this is as simple as rocking from side to side.

What else will help?

Inflammatory substances are like glue and they adhese muscle fibres together, which reduces mobility. Anti-inflammatory drugs, such as aspirin, are good for relieving the pain. If you don't like taking medication, herbs such as devil's claw and turmeric have anti-inflammatory qualities. You should also apply ice to the injured area, for example using a bag of frozen peas. If you ever watch a sports physiotherapist tending a sporting injury on the pitch or field, one of the first things they will do is apply an ice pack to the affected area. This prevents inflammatory substances from entering the tissue and speeds recovery. Never place ice directly on the skin – wrap it in a cloth first. Keep it in position for ten minutes and then repeat the process an hour later. It is best not to apply heat during the first twenty-four hours.

DAY TWO

Your back may start to feel more bruised than painful – a good sign that it's beginning to heal. You must still take it easy, though you should try to walk around a bit to stimulate circulation. Always listen to your body, as it is invariably telling you something useful. Some types of back pain (usually muscular) may start to feel better with gentle movement but others (usually nerve types) will hurt more. If you find the pain gets worse as you move about, then be sensible and go back to bed.

DAY THREE

This is D-Day as regards the seriousness of the problem. If the intensity of the symptoms is decreasing, it's very likely that your back is regulating itself and there should be no need to see a specialist. If you are on the road to recovery and you now have an ache rather than a pain, you can start treating yourself with heat rather than ice (see page 33).

If, however, the pain feels worse or you can detect that it has moved to the limbs (referral symptoms), you should contact an osteopath or similar specialist immediately.

Emergency hug

Doing exercises during an acute phase of back pain is generally unwise, but the hug shown on page 100 is particularly gentle and often very soothing for most types of back pain. Back pain is often caused by the joints and soft tissues being squashed together. This hug works by opening up the vertebrae in your lower back and stimulating blood flow to the muscles in this area. Most people should find it gives relief. If it doesn't, allow more time for the area to settle and ask your therapist whether it is a suitable exercise for your injury.

PAINKILLERS

Drugs are very effective at pain relief particularly in the short term. (For long-term use and possible side effects see pages 76 and 79.) If the pain is not too severe, take a paracetamol-based drug, which has no side effect on the stomach. Alternatively, you could buy a pain-relief patch to provide a local painkilling effect at the site of the pain (the drug enters the bloodstream without going via the liver, meaning that it works more quickly and there is no risk of liver damage). The most powerful over-the-counter painkiller/anti-inflammatory drugs contain a mixture of ibuprofen (aspirin-based) and codeine. Be aware, however, that codeine can cause constipation, which sometimes makes back pain worse.

HEAT AND ICE

Changing the temperature of the skin can help moderate the processing of the pain sensations in the spinal cord, which is why there are so many pain-relieving products that utilize this method. When muscles go into spasm because of injury, both heat and ice can be used to desensitize the nerve endings. Different types of back pain respond to different temperatures.

Cooling usually works best on acute injuries and nerve pain as it helps reduce inflammation. If it's a muscular strain, heat is usually the most effective, but you should still use ice for the first twenty-four hours. To use heat, place a hot-water bottle against the most painful part of your back. Alternatively, if the pain is not too severe, soaking in a hot bath may help, but you don't want to get yourself in a situation where you get struck by severe pain as you try to get out again. In addition you can buy special ice packs (which can also be heated), as well as heat patches that increase the skin temperature, from mail-order companies, chemists or back-care shops.

The power of heat

Mary, 26, designer

The problem

Some people may notice that their back pain gets worse in cold, wind or damp conditions.

The solution

Heat will generally help. A hot bath/shower, heat patch or heat rub can all be effective.

I have a chronic upper-back problem, which means I spend most of my life doubled up from pain in my shoulder and neck. Over the years I've tried to find ways to help myself deal with the pain. The cold definitely exacerbates it so I try to avoid going out or working in an air-conditioned office. I sleep with a hot-water bottle under the sore area, which seems to work. Taking a hot shower and letting the water trickle down my shoulder is nice. Sometimes going for a walk helps me switch off from the pain, too.

Garry says: Having recently travelled to Nordic countries to witness their extensive use of sauna, hot water and steam, I strongly believe these heat treatments can be of tremendous benefit to anyone with muscular aches and pains, particularly when they notice that pain gets worse in cold, wind or damp conditions. If you are in the fortunate position of being able to afford a hot tub or Jacuzzi, this is an excellent way of counteracting the effects of stresses and strains on the muscular system. Otherwise just take a hot bath or shower.

MASSAGE

The Greek physician Hippocrates believed that massage was the mother of all therapies and that was more than a thousand years ago. The principle still holds true today, particularly with regard to back pain. Massage is a useful technique for improving circulation, which can help relieve pain and tension. The sort of massage on offer in a beauty salon is often very superficial and more like a skin polish; the type you need for muscular pain and tension reaches far deeper, allowing the therapist to locate the exact site of pain and work on relieving any muscular tension there.

You don't need to be a skilled practitioner in order to give a good massage – it is actually a very instinctive skill. If you knock yourself you automatically rub the area to make it feel better, which is exactly what a massage does. A daily shoulder massage does wonders to relieve tension and relax the back. Why not strike a deal with your partner that you'll both spend a few minutes each day massaging each other's shoulders? Although in theory you could massage yourself, it is so much nicer having someone else do it for you – a 'treat' meant (treatment) for you! Learning to give a good

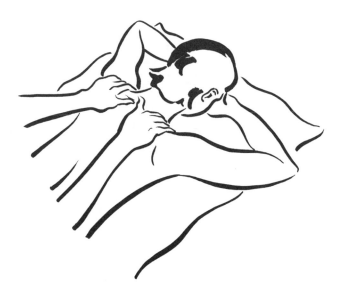

Muscular tension

Tom, 41, actor and writer

The problem
Muscular tension is a common problem and can lead to back pain.

The solution
Regular massage is one way to relieve muscular tension in the back. Stretching can also help.

I am a big believer in massage as I've found this has really helped me cope with a lifetime of back problems that go back to my school days when I played football and rugby. Over the years I've tried different masseurs all over the world. I regularly treat myself to a massage as this helps loosen up my spine when my back is not feeling spot-on. I've had a few back problems simply through wear and tear. What usually happens is that I pull a muscle in the spine. It's not the sort of pain that's excruciating but it does cause discomfort and restricts my movement. If you are susceptible to back problems like I am, it is really important to look after your spine or it will just get worse. Regular massages really do seem to help.

Garry says: I believe that good massage should be the cornerstone of any physical therapy clinic. It is such a tried-and-tested technique for muscle tension. It is also excellent for promoting relaxation, self-healing and detoxification. For the sake of a healthy back you need a deep-tissue massage that isolates the areas of tension and then releases them. A recent study suggested that acupressure massage was one of the best techniques for the treatment of back pain. It can be a little bit painful but it is highly beneficial in the long run.

massage is not that difficult – most people have an intuitive feel for it. All that is required is confidence.

When it's your turn to play masseur, close your eyes and allow your fingers to lead you to the points of tension. Ask your partner for feedback to the bits that hurt. When you find a tender area, apply gentle pressure there for a few seconds, then release, kneading with thumbs and fingers.

Although it's not quite as enjoyable, you can also massage yourself by squeezing the tops of your shoulders with your fingers or massaging down the sides of your neck with both hands. Alternatively, you could invest in a hand-held massage machine. Although this can never replace the sensitivity of human hands, it can be a good way to boost circulation, which is one of the main aims of massage.

Summary

- Don't panic! Most cases of back pain show signs of improvement in three days.

- There is a lot you can do to treat yourself – ice, heat and over-the-counter drugs may be all you need to get through it.

- Massage is a good way to relax the muscles and prevent pain.

CHAPTER 3

Defining pain

One of the scariest things about back pain is feeling in the dark and not understanding what is going on. If your symptoms have not subsided after three days, it is always best to consult a professional, both for reassurance and to make sure you get the right treatment straight away. If you have never suffered from back pain before, your first port of call should be your GP, to rule out any other medical cause as much as anything. You will be asked to describe your back pain and to do a series of tests, such as bending forwards and checking your reflexes, in order that your GP can a get a truer picture of the cause of pain. The GP will give you a thorough physical examination and should be able to make a preliminary diagnosis. You may be recommended more bed rest and prescribed painkillers, anti-inflammatory drugs and muscle relaxants.

If the problem is very severe or does not clear up, the doctor may refer you to an osteopath, chiropractor or physiotherapist for treatment (see page 53 for an explanation of the differences) or send you for further tests such as an MRI scan (see page 66), which will show exactly what damage has been done.

The first time you visit a specialist practitioner, you will be asked some fairly standard questions to help lead the practitioner to an initial diagnosis. Your history will provide an idea of what structure is likely to be involved. This will be followed by a physical examination, stressing the individual structure that seems to be at the root of the problem. For example, if you stretch a ligament and the pain is exacerbated, this is physical proof that it is the ligament that is the problem. If there is no pain when the ligament is stretched, the practitioner will rule out ligament involvement and need to check other structures, such as a disc (by compressing it) or a muscle (by simply moving it).

Avoid the temptation to try to diagnose your own back problem: even practitioners with decades of clinical experience would not attempt to do so without examining you carefully. It is worth, however, considering the questions below. At the very least they will help you prepare for your session with the practitioner and may also help you understand a bit more about what is going on with your back. Take the answers with you to your first appointment.

HOW BAD IS THE PAIN?

Pain is very subjective: what feels unbearable for one person may be perceived as a mild ache for another. It is a good idea to keep a personal pain chart, rating your pain on a daily basis from nought to ten.

HOW DID IT COME ON?

This is a key question, as it will give the practitioner an indication of what structures may be involved. The following will be common answers to this question.

Strenuous or unaccustomed exercise

If this is your answer and the pain came on immediately after doing any of these physical activities, there is a good chance that this sort of back pain is a muscular problem and will often subside within a few days.

Bending down to pick something up or lifting a heavy weight

Ligament pain often comes on through prolonged stretching in any direction (forwards, backwards, sideways). This sort of pain is often eased when lying still or resting.

No obvious cause

If the pain has just crept up on you, the problem may not just be mechanical. Your practitioner will want to know all about your medical history and whether you are currently or have recently been on any medication. You will probably be asked if you have lost weight, have a fever, sleep problems or any other unusual symptoms in order to rule out any underlying problems.

The pain really started after twenty-four hours

Being unaware of the problem at first, then really beginning to notice it twenty-four hours after an injury is a common pattern with a disc problem. It is not until the disc swells or ruptures that it compresses the nerve and pain comes on. This can take a day or so to kick in.

HOW OLD ARE YOU?

Age is very relevant in terms of back pain. At each stage of the ageing process you become more prone to certain back problems. By the age of seventy, the skeleton of an average person is about a third lighter than it was at forty.

Telling the practitioner how old you are can help pinpoint what may be causing your pain, so don't be bashful about your age. For example, if you are over forty, it could be the initial signs of osteoarthritis (wear and tear). This can affect isolated joints in the body such as ankles, knees or hips as well as the spine. Rheumatoid arthritis often attacks many joints, not just one, and is not necessarily associated with age. (See also page 27.)

Osteoporosis (brittle-bone disease) commonly affects women over the age of fifty. It is particularly important to make your practitioner aware if you know you have this condition, as any manual therapy techniques will need to be lighter and more sensitive to your skeleton's needs.

Balance also deteriorates with age and a simple fall can prove disastrous, particularly if you are overweight or have osteoporosis. (For more on pain and age, see chapter 11, pages 174–86.)

WHAT SORT OF PAIN IS IT?

Pain manifests itself in a variety of ways. Aggravating factors will often indicate whether further tests will be needed.

General aches
This is another sign of osteoarthritis, sometimes aggravated by cold and damp weather. You may need x-rays for confirmation.

Sharp, shooting, burning pain
Such pain could be caused by many things, including muscular tears or nerve compression.

Tingling, numbness or pins and needles
All these symptoms will refer into the limbs and indicate that there must be nerve involvement as this is the only structure to cause this change in sensation.

CASE HISTORY ⑥

Exacerbating the pain

Pete, 48, football club chairman

The problem
Fear can be another aggravating factor in back pain as it can cause muscular tension and make you more aware of the pain.

The solution
Don't be scared to get a diagnosis. The relief of knowing what the problem is can be immense. Once you have a positive diagnosis, an appropriate action plan can be devised.

There have been times that the pain in my back has been so bad I can hardly move. On one particularly scary occasion I could hardly breathe and thought I was having a heart attack. Fortunately, these attacks have been short-lived and once I get to see Garry it normally clears up quickly. The fear of what is happening is often worse than the pain itself.

Anything can trigger it, such as coughing or bending over to tie a shoelace. The problem for me is that the nerves have been damaged since I had shingles as a child. It left me with a numb hip so I don't realize when I'm doing something that puts my back at risk.

Garry says: Sometimes people who go to A&E departments thinking they are having a heart attack actually have a trapped nerve in the thoracic spine. This can be very frightening and it is obviously important that any chest pain is explored medically. (Someone once said that if there was an osteopath in each A&E department, he or she could quickly evaluate whether there was a musculoskeletal origin to the pain.)

The nerve supply to the whole body comes via your back. Every vertebra has a set of nerves and wherever these connect symptoms can arise. Nerves in the neck can refer pain into the arms; nerves in the lower back can refer pain into the legs (e.g. sciatica); nerves in the mid-back can refer to the chest.

It is unfortunate for Pete that he has nerve damage as this means he does not get the usual warning signals when pain is starting to build up. Thankfully, Pete responds very well to treatment and over the last twenty years several acute episodes have been controlled with treatment.

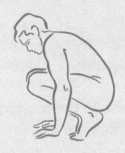

HOW LONG HAVE YOU BEEN IN PAIN?

The duration of the pain is a good predictor as to whether this problem is something likely to heal by itself or whether more treatment and investigation is needed. If the area starts to feel more bruised than painful within the first twenty-four hours, the chances are that you are on the mend and will not need treatment.

If the pain is starting to get worse by day three, it could be a disc problem or another unrelated health issue. Professional help is very important in these situations.

WHAT IS THE PATTERN TO YOUR PAIN?

How and when you have symptoms can tell a practitioner a lot about your back problem. Try to keep a diary of symptoms in order to give an accurate appraisal.

Better at night, worse in the morning

This suggests that the problem is most likely muscular because an increase in circulation from all the movement in the day has eased the muscles. The practitioner may also want to know if heat relieves your pain. If the problem is muscular, the answer is likely to be yes because heat increases circulation. You will also be asked if movement aggravates the pain or not. With extreme muscular strains, any movement can initially feel agonizing, but gentle movement/mobilization usually eases the situation, again because it increases blood flow.

Better in the morning, worse as the day progresses

This could indicate a nerve problem. When still and non-aggravated, symptoms tend to be minimal. Movement can aggravate the sensitive nerves. If it is a nerve problem, your body is likely to have gone into spasm, as this is the body's way of protecting the nerve and more sensitive underlying structures from further damage. If it is a disc problem, the pain may also be more intense at night as the discs will have lost a bit of height over the course of the day. When you lie flat the discs rehydrate, which can put a bit of pressure on areas of inflammation.

Are you in pain even when not moving?
This may be something serious. Mechanical pain usually settles down when you are still. If you are in pain all the time, even when not moving, you may need further investigation.

HAVE YOU HAD THIS SORT OF PAIN BEFORE?

This may be relevant. The practitioner will also want to know what treatment you have had in the past, with what success and whether you have consulted your doctor. You may also be asked about your family history – some people will have a genetic predisposition to certain conditions. And, of course, it is very important to mention if you are pregnant. Pregnancy produces the hormone relaxin, which softens all the ligaments in the body, including those in the back. (See also pages 176–79.)

DO YOU HAVE ANY OTHER SYMPTOMS?

All physical therapists must be aware of what are known as the 'red flag signs'. They may ask if you have had other symptoms, such as nausea, loss of appetite, weight loss, night sweats, chest or stomach pain, dizziness, headaches, tingling or numbness in the limbs. These may just be symptoms of referred pain but your practitioner will need to be able to rule out that they do not indicate anything more serious. Proper diagnosis is essential to good practice.

CASE HISTORY ❼

Mystery cause

Harry, 48, designer

The problem
A side effect of medication.

The solution
Always tell your GP or practitioner what other medications you are on as this may be relevant to the diagnosis.

My story is quite strange. I was very fit and used to jog for three to four miles each day with my dog. Then suddenly I found myself feeling totally exhausted by this and got terrible pains in my legs. I was also getting backache. I went to see my GP who sent me to an orthopaedic surgeon. They ran all sorts of tests on me, including an MRI scan, and I went to other specialists, too. For several weeks no one could discover what was causing the symptoms.

Eventually one of the specialists made a connection with some tablets I had been taking for a few months for a stomach ailment called colitis. It was apparently unusual but it had affected the muscles in my legs and that was why I was in pain. I came off the tablets but the pain remained for several months as I think the medicine must have still been in my bloodstream. Throughout this period, I managed the pain with acupuncture. But the biggest relief was finding the cause.

Garry says: Nearly all medications come with side effects and if you suddenly develop strange symptoms or pain it is always worth checking first of all whether there is a link or not.

Harry's backache was caused from the problem in his legs. The way he was walking had put his whole back out of alignment.

It is a big myth that an osteopath just treats the back. Osteopaths are trained in treating the whole body and know how to look at ergonomics, lifestyle and diet. Most medications have side effects and should be considered when trying to establish a positive diagnosis. This is why it is good for osteopaths to work in conjunction with doctors rather than in isolation. The fuller the picture you can paint, the better the outcome.

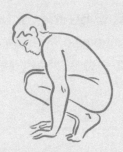

The following are examples of questions you may be asked:

Do you have a temperature or pain just above your waist?
A temperature of 38°C (100°F) or more and pain in the back just above the waist can indicate pyelonephritis, a kidney inflammation usually caused by a bacterial infection. There may be some urinary symptoms too. It is important to see your doctor immediately.

When any internal organ, such as the lungs, liver, spleen, heart, stomach or kidneys, is not working properly, symptoms can arise in the back. For example, back pain with urinary symptoms can be a sign of an enlarged prostate gland, particularly in men over fifty years old. If a practitioner suspects that an organ is involved, they should refer to your GP.

Do you have any loss of bladder or bowel control?
This suggests a severe nerve compression and it is likely you will need surgery. This is certainly a case to go to the emergency room of your nearest hospital.

Summary

- Keep a pain diary, noting down when and where you experience symptoms and how long they last.

- Answer the questions in this chapter carefully and take them with you if you go to see a doctor or practitioner.

- The more information you take with you, the better.

- Don't try to diagnose the problem yourself. Sometimes the fear of what might be wrong can actually aggravate the problem.

CHAPTER 4

Getting professional help

As discussed on page 38, if your symptoms continue for more than three days you should visit your GP for a physical examination and preliminary diagnosis. You may then need to visit a specialist for further treatment. This will most often be an osteopath, chiropractor or physiotherapist, but other treatments may sometimes be necessary.

MANIPULATIVE TREATMENTS

Manipulative therapy is an age-old technique. The principle is to release any normally mobile joints that have got stuck. The patient needs to be positioned so that the vertebra is isolated and then a short thrusting motion can be applied to release it. Practitioners used to be referred to as 'bone setters'. The underlying principle for all these treatments is to lubricate the surfaces of the joints in order to restore mobility. Manipulative therapies incorporate massage and mobilization to the soft tissues as well as a short sharp thrust, applied so that the stretch goes through to the underlying joint.

In need of an MOT

Richard, 40, marketing director in the music industry

The problem
Back pain is often due to an accumulation of tensions – a case of the straw that breaks the camel's back.

The solution
People who are prone to back pain or feel symptoms coming on should go for regular check-ups just as they would go to the dentist or take their car in for an MOT.

From my late twenties onwards, I seem to have had a series of aches and pains in my back. There has never been any specific pattern. Sometimes it's my lower back, at other times it's the middle and sometimes it's my upper back and shoulders. The first couple of practitioners I saw really didn't seem to do me any good – one just gave me a very rough massage, while the other tried to realign me but did nothing to help the pain.

I started seeing Garry about a year ago and go on a regular basis about once a month. It is really just maintenance work but it's still very important as whatever the problem is he seems to be able to correct it and prevent it from getting worse. He's also given me lots of good advice on posture and lifestyle, which has finally sunk in so that I now consciously try to sit better at a computer.

In my case, I think my back is just not very robust and needs to be regularly knocked into shape.

Garry says: Most of us don't think twice about regular check-ups at the dentist. For someone like Richard, regular back check-ups have also proved valuable. Some back pains are accumulative in nature and, in much the same way as a valve needs to be released on a pressure cooker, need to be dealt with before the problem builds up to become chronic and debilitating. Some people frown at the thought of spending money to maintain their health, yet don't think twice about spending money to destroy it.

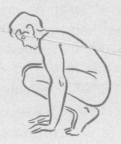

CHOOSING A THERAPIST

One of the hardest things about having back pain can be knowing who to go to for help. Ask your GP for a recommendation or find out from friends who they have seen. If a name crops up a few times, the chances are they are good. If you have no point of referral, contact one of the associations listed at the end of this book (see pages 189–90).

When you go to a therapist for the first time, use your instincts. Do you feel relaxed in their care? Do you feel they are giving you enough time and attention? Beware of anyone who tries to sign you up for long courses of treatment – therapists should re-evaluate their patients' progress and treatment after about every three sessions. Never be scared to ask questions – good practitioners should not cloak what they do in mystery.

There are many alternative treatments that require only minimal training, sometimes as little as a weekend. These should not be confused or compared with mainstream treatments such as osteopathy and physiotherapy, which require years of training. Longer courses will teach therapists not only what they can treat but also, and more importantly, what they can't. Good therapists should refer you on to someone else with more relevant expertise when they know they cannot help rather than just leave you floundering. Never be embarrassed to ask the therapist about their training or to see proof of membership of a professional association. Finally, beware of therapists who have too much to say for themselves – they may be trying to lull you into a false sense of security. The treatment should speak for itself not the therapist.

OSTEOPATHY AND CHIROPRACTIC

Some practitioners get very worked up about it, but the truth is that the differences between osteopathy and chiropractic are slight. Indeed, most osteopaths and chiropractors would be hard-pressed to explain them. As a general rule, chiropractors use more x-rays, particularly for diagnosis. Osteopaths are more cautious about using x-rays, believing that the information thereby obtained is minimal compared to the inherent risk of radiation.

Osteopathy

Osteopathy was pioneered in 1874 by the American Andrew Taylor Still. It is a system of manual treatment to the spine and other parts of the body. Osteopathy looks at back pain in relation to the whole spine, pelvis, lower limbs and muscle imbalance. Qualified osteopaths in the UK spend five years training in anatomy, physiology, biochemistry and clinical examination and treatment of muscular and skeletal disorders. Osteopathy and medicine have a lot in common. They both use scientific knowledge of anatomy and physiology and clinical methods of investigation. An osteopath knows enough about pathology to recognize conditions that should be referred to a medically qualified practitioner.

Osteopathy used to be considered an 'alternative' medicine, working independently of the mainstream. It has gradually been integrated into the UK health system, becoming a complementary medicine. Osteopathy and chiropractic are now recognized by the government, which means you should be able to get treatment covered by medical insurance companies. Whereas the old osteopath used no medicine whatsoever, the modern practitioner recognizes the benefits and requirements in certain cases of medical intervention. It has been suggested that in the future osteopaths may be given some rights to prescribe medications to their patients although this is not yet in force.

CASE HISTORY ❾

Finding a therapist

Ben, 34, architectural designer

The problem
Back pain is such a common problem that sometimes it can seem that every alternative therapist on the high street is offering his or her services.

The solution
Recommendation is good, but follow your own instincts, too. Read up on how the therapy works on the following pages and don't be afraid to ask questions.

One of the worst things about back pain – probably worse even than the pain itself – is that everyone you meet is such a know-it-all and tells you what to do about it or who to see. My back problems started when I was knocked off my Vespa moped in 2004. It was quite a nasty accident and it took me a long time to recover. Eight months later I was left with chronic pain in my lower back and a shooting, stabbing pain down my right leg.

I went to see an osteopath in Harley Street who told me he thought it was related to the moped accident – not a strenuous bout of gardening, which I had originally blamed. He also explained that the shooting pain down my leg was sciatica caused by a trapped nerve. Although his diagnosis was good, I didn't really take to that particular osteopath – his prices were extortionate and the treatment room dirty. Relieved to know why I was in pain, I decided to just leave it for a while as I was going on holiday.

The pain, however, got worse and worse and on a couple of occasions I found I could not even get out of bed. As I had to travel to the States for six weeks for work, I went to my GP for help. My GP gave me an anti-inflammatory drug, which really did the trick and meant I could get on that plane. When I came back to the UK I was feeling really low and debilitated. All my friends started bombarding me with recommendations of practitioners they knew.

Eventually someone recommended Garry. As soon as I walked into his clinic, I knew this was the sort of place I wanted to be treated. The treatments took a while to work. I've now done about five sessions and have managed to come off the anti-inflammatories, which was my main goal. Life is slowly getting back to normal again. I can walk to work and will soon be able to exercise again. I'm so glad to be where I am now – living with continual nagging pain is really stressful. As was finding the right person to help.

Garry says: Recommendation is the best way to source a good practitioner – if someone's name comes up twice, take note of it, but try not to get bombarded with other people's well-meaning advice. What is right for one person may not be right for you. It's good to explore or experiment as to what suits your needs. And, of course, it is right and proper to consult your GP so that he or she can rule out any other possibilities.

Remember that the principle of treatment is to get better, not to become someone's regular, so beware of anyone who suggests lengthy courses of treatment.

Ben is now at a stage when the pain is beginning to subside. This is a good time to introduce mobility techniques (stretching). Once he has regained his range of movement he will be able to start doing some strengthening exercises. He is now off all medication and is improving well.

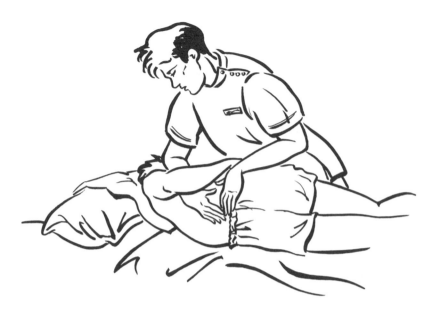

The underlying principle in osteopathy is that structure governs function. Correct structure should allow unimpaired nerve and blood supply to all areas of the body. An osteopath uses techniques such as stretching the soft tissues around the joint to bring back the total range of movement. An osteopath may well give advice on ergonomics, something that most conventional doctors might not link to back pain, and can advise on the impact of posture, lifestyle and stress.

Check that your osteopath is a member of the appropriate body, such as the General Osteopathic Council in the UK. This ensures that they have been carefully vetted and adhere to the desired standard of training and codes of practice. Members of the Council also have to undertake at least thirty hours of continuing professional development annually. The General Osteopathic Council can provide details of the nearest qualified osteopath to where you live.

Chiropractic

The first chiropractic treatment was given in 1895 by the American Daniel David Palmer. Although he was jailed the following year for practising without a licence, today thousands of people, particularly back pain sufferers, are helped by his manipulative techniques.

The word 'chiropractic' comes from the classical Greek 'chieri' (meaning hand) and 'praktikos' (meaning performed). Chiropractors specialize in the diagnosis, treatment and prevention of bio-mechanical disorders of the musculoskeletal system, particularly those involving the spine and their effects on the nervous system.

Like osteopathy, chiropractic is very successful in treating back pain. It consists of a wide range of specific manual techniques designed to improve the function of joints, relieve pain and muscle spasm and irritation to the nervous system. Chiropractic treatment also works well for neck pain, arm pain and headaches. In the UK, the British Chiropractic Association can help you find a nearby practitioner.

Going for treatment

Many osteopaths and chiropractors work in short treatment courses so that they can continually re-evaluate how you're doing. They will be looking to see how you have responded to the last treatment and how well the natural healing process is working. If treatment does not seem to be having a positive effect, they may try something different. As the natural healing process kicks in, they will be able to give slightly different treatments. For example, they cannot give high-velocity thrusts when the body is locked in spasm, but once you are very nearly better, a treatment like this could set you on the path to total recovery.

What is the crack?

Techniques of treatment between practitioners vary greatly but will involve gentle manipulation and soft tissue work. A common cause of back pain is a joint becoming stuck (see also page 26). If this is the case, 'cracking' the joint can bring instant relief. Don't be alarmed if you hear clicks or cracking sounds as the joint surfaces are moved apart. This is quite normal and should not hurt. A common misconception regarding manipulation is that something has gone 'out' and needs to be put back in, whereas actually the joint has got stuck and needs to be released. Looking at it this way makes it sound less dramatic! There is far more to manipulation, however, than just getting a click, so don't worry if your treatment is silent.

Will it hurt?

Treatment itself is not usually painful, unless the practitioner really homes in on the source of pain. Bear in mind that any pain you experience during treatment is likely to be nothing compared to the pain you are probably already suffering. Therefore, it really is worth grinning and bearing it because with treatment you are more likely to get better faster. Sometimes there is pain after treatment with symptoms getting worse before they get better. You will normally be asked to go back for another treatment and an assessment about three days after your first treatment. If symptoms have not started to ease off, the practitioner may decide to take a different approach. A good practitioner should be continually re-assessing treatment in relation to how your body is responding.

Too scared to go for treatment

Jane, 41, record producer

The problem
Many people are terrified of having their neck cracked.

The solution
Go to someone you trust for treatment. Explain to them beforehand your fears; they may be able to do the treatment without cracking.

I've always had a phobia about my neck being crunched so this was the worst hurdle to overcome in my treatment after a skiing accident in Meribel. The accident was stupid: I was a complete novice and just going too fast. My skis tripped over my sticks and I took a huge fall, landing on my shoulder and then bouncing across the piste. When I picked myself up again, I thought, OK, I'm fine. I even managed to ski down to the bottom of the piste. It must have been adrenalin because a couple of hours afterwards I started to seize up. The pain began in my neck and was so overwhelming I couldn't tell at that point that my back, leg and thumb were hurt as well. I went to the medical centre in the resort where they x-rayed my back and said that the top four vertebrae had been pushed together. They gave me lots of painkillers and anti-inflammatory drugs and put my neck in a brace, which they said I needed to wear for ten days. I was also advised to see a physiotherapist every day.

I did not feel fit enough to travel straightaway so I spent a boring few days trying to recuperate in the resort. The physio was not very successful as I was in so much pain, I could not bear to be touched, so there was little that they could do. When I got back home I went straight to see Garry, who I had been to see once before just to loosen up my shoulders with a massage. I told him about my phobia with my neck. He was very calm and gentle and helped coax me through it all.

Garry says: It's quite common and understandable to have a phobia about having your neck cracked. It's an area that is very sensitive as it is so rich in nerve supply. I think people have just seen too many torture scenes in movies involving the neck being snapped. This is not what osteopathy manipulation is about! Admittedly, it does look and sound somewhat extreme, but it would not be performed unless it was of therapeutic value.

The sound you hear when you crack a joint is caused by the joint surfaces gapping. This causes a carbon dioxide release resulting in an implosion of synovial fluid (natural lubricant) onto the joint's surfaces, which eases the joints. Sometimes if you just turn or move, you might hear your joints click or ping. When an osteopath releases a stuck joint surface by manipulation the sound is usually more like a thud. It can provide instant relief.

The medical centre told Jane that her top four vertebrae had been compressed. This is actually the most painful thing to happen to the vertebrae because it can cause pain on both sides of the spine, whereas in other types of injury the vertebrae twist in a rotational direction. Traction is the best technique for treating compression. This is something that a practitioner will provide during a treatment, usually by cupping their hands behind the base of your skull and gently and slowly leaning backwards, producing a mild, elongating stretch along the neck. Alternatively, you can buy weighted traction devices that hang from the door, which cradle under the chin and the base of the skull. Jane was given a brace, which both provided mild traction and helped immobilize the area. Braces are commonly issued for neck injuries, especially where movement is the aggravating factor.

Jane noticed that her body was in too much pain for a physio to be able to help her. The body lets you do only what is right for it at that moment. There is a self-healing process going on within the body and treatment should assist and speed this process up. The job of a practitioner is to assess how far this self-healing process has progressed and apply appropriate techniques for that stage. For example, many manipulative techniques will be out of the question if a patient is doubled up with pain. Some patients have come to me in so much pain that I can hardly touch them. Acupuncture can be the best solution in such a scenario (see pages 63–64).

Jane has grown in confidence with each treatment and I am pleased to see tremendous improvement in the injury as well as a lifting of her spirits as the pain has gone.

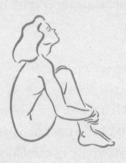

PHYSIOTHERAPY

Doctors often refer patients to physiotherapists as they both share a medical background. Physiotherapy is fantastic for restoring muscle function after injury or surgery. A lot of physiotherapists are employed in hospitals, where patients are bed bound and need physical stimulation.

In many ways, physiotherapy is much like osteopathy or chiropractic, but it is less 'hands-on' than either of these physical therapies. It also uses various electrical treatments, which stimulate the deeper tissues to encourage drainage and the dispersal of inflammatory waste products. An infrared lamp is often used to provide heat to help the muscles relax. A physiotherapist is also skilled at simple massage and mobilization and, like an osteopath or chiropractor, will take time to observe the way you walk, stand, sit, bend, etc. You will probably also be prescribed specific exercises to speed recovery.

ACUPUNCTURE

Acupuncture has been a major form of medicine in China for 5000 years and can be one of the best drug-free ways to relieve pain. It relaxes the nervous system by controlling the central pain pathways and also promotes the release of the body's own pain-relieving hormones, endorphins. Endorphins have almost the same chemical structure as morphine. The release of endorphins can now be scientifically measured by taking a sample of spinal fluid before and after treatment. New research has also shown that acupuncture can activate a part of the brain called the 'limbic brain', which modulates and eases the perception of pain. This mimics what drugs are supposed to do for pain relief but without taking drugs.

Chinese medicine is based on the principle of a life force ('chi') or energy that passes through the body. There can be too much, too little or a blockage of 'chi'. The aim of Chinese medicine is to correct any imbalance in this life force, as this is seen as the cause of disharmony or disease, and to allow the body's natural healing mechanisms to do the rest. The Chinese regard good health as a state of energy balance within the body.

The principle of all physical therapy is to improve the blood supply to the affected area in order to promote healing, which is exactly what acupuncture does. When a fine needle or any foreign body is inserted into the skin, it stimulates the body's defence system to send extra blood to the area to fight off potential infection. When treating back pain, the needles are inserted into the area of pain, as well as into specific acupuncture points, as this extra blood supply reduces muscular spasm, pain and inflammation. Acupuncture can make the ensuing manipulation and mobilization work much easier and patients are always surprised by how relaxed it makes them feel – and it has none of the nasty side effects that go hand in hand with muscle-relaxant drugs. Because it's so gentle, acupuncture is also an ideal treatment choice for the elderly.

IF THE PAIN DOES NOT GET BETTER

The back is generally good at healing itself and any treatment such as osteopathy is usually just speeding this process along. Occasionally, even with treatment, the back takes a long time to heal, in which case you may need to consider some alternative.

Spinal injections

If your pain is very severe and none of the conventional treatments seem to help, you may be recommended to have a spinal injection to counteract the inflammation. A dose of cortico-steroid (a powerful anti-inflammatory) is injected into the nerve root and the

Needle phobia

Martha, 32, designer

The problem

A phobia of needles is common and often related to a bad experience with injections or blood tests.

The solution

If you have a needle phobia, tell your practitioner; they may be able to reassure you. But if you really cannot bear the thought of needles there are many alternatives, including acupressure (finger pressure) and electrotherapy devices.

I've always been scared of needles so was very unsure when I was offered acupuncture on my back. It probably helped that I was lying face down and couldn't see what was being done. I was in so much pain with my back anyway that anything that could help with this seemed worth trying. I must admit I did cringe every time a needle went in but that was purely because of the idea of it. About half a dozen were used in total but it wasn't painful at all and I actually loved the sensation – I could really feel a rush of blood around the area where the needle was inserted. It seemed to immediately distract me from the pain. Afterwards I felt as if I'd had a couple of glasses of wine. It is nothing like having an injection or blood test. The needle doesn't feel as though it's going in very far and the whole process is actually very pleasurable.

Garry says: The insertion of fine needles is usually painless, though it sometimes produces a mild stinging sensation for a second or two. Disposable needles are used to prevent cross-infection. Once they are in place, they are left for about fifteen minutes. Usually the acupuncturist will twiddle the needles to adjust the energy flow. If you are needle-phobic, there are other ways to stimulate the acupressure points – through laser, electrical, heat or finger pressure.

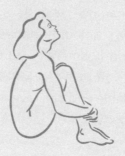

affected spinal joint. Alternatively, an epidural injection may be given to combine the benefits of local anaesthetic and cortisone. Sometimes with an epidural the pain gets worse for a day or two before it starts taking effect. Spinal injections are often used to reduce symptoms. If they fail then surgery will often follow.

X-rays and scans

If your back pain is not improving you may be recommended an x-ray or MRI scan. An x-ray is good at showing bones, while an MRI (multi-resonance imaging) scan is a much more expensive technique that shows not only bones, but also nerves, discs, tendons, muscles and ligaments – all the structures that could possibly be causing you pain. An MRI scan is probably the best diagnostic scan available and can give a three-dimensional image of the inside of the body.

Surgery

Surgery is usually used as a very last resort. Less than ten per cent of back problems lead to an operation – the most common one requiring surgery is a prolapsed, ruptured or slipped disc. This is when the soft pulpy nucleus of the disc squirts out through a tear in the disc's outer edge.. The idea of a surgical operation on the spine can be very alarming but techniques have improved considerably and often use microsurgery, which is much less invasive as well as more successful.

Microsurgery involves passing a fibre-optic camera through a small incision down to where the disc protrudes. The surgeon can see exactly what he is doing on a screen. A small 'snipper' (trimming instrument) is then introduced through the incision down to the offending disc. After the protrusion has been trimmed, a small suction cleaner is inserted to remove any remaining disc fragments. Once the operation is complete, only one stitch is required to close the incision site.

CASE HISTORY ⑫

Disc surgery

Nick, 47, advertising executive

The problem
Accumulation of stresses, such as running on hard ground, lack of stretching, poor muscle tone and bad posture can eventually take their toll and cause a disc to weaken, then rupture.

The solution
If the problem is severe, surgery may be the only alternative.

I've had the odd twinge of back pain in the past but no history of any consequence. It all started when I went for a run one morning. I'd bought a brand new pair of running shoes but they felt strange, as though there was too much cushioning – completely different to how they had felt when I had tried them on in the shop. I also noticed during the run that there was a lot more compressive force than usual travelling through my back.

When I got back home I did some sit-ups, had a hot bath and stretched. Later that day I went to work and everything seemed fine. I asked my colleague how her back was doing, as she had been having pain. As I said this, I stretched out to reach for the mouse on my computer and my own back went into spasm. I've never experienced anything like it. It was like having a vice around my midriff – I was totally locked and couldn't move. It was so embarrassing as I started to sweat profusely and within seconds my shirt was soaked. I told my secretary to cancel all my meetings – quite something for a self-confessed workaholic! But there was no way I could even move.

Getting home was incredibly difficult. As soon as I was back in my apartment I lay down on the living room floor. Instinctively I knew I should lie flat with no movement. Even the smallest movement sent excruciating waves of pain through me. I knew Garry socially so I phoned him in a panic from the floor. He advised me to stay lying flat, take anti-inflammatories, get someone to apply an ice pack on the painful area and then to make contact with him again in the morning.

Being self-employed, I forced myself to get back into work the next day. As long as I kept completely still, the pain was tolerable. Moving or getting up from a chair, however, was agonizing. That evening I went out for dinner and could feel myself locking up even more. The pain was getting worse not better. During the night it started to move down my left leg and by the morning I had numbness and pins and needles below the knee. I immediately phoned Garry who said I should go in to see him as soon as possible.

When he examined me he said my knee reflex had disappeared, suggesting it could be a disc problem. He gave me some acupuncture, which helped a little with the pain, and recommended that I had an MRI scan. That night I almost cried myself to sleep, as the pain was particularly bad at night.

When I had the MRI the next day, they found a large disc protrusion, which was compressing the nerve that went down the front of my leg. This apparently explained the pain, loss of sensation and lack of reflex.

Much to my dismay, Garry said I was now beyond the realms of physical therapy and needed to see a surgeon. As my brother had back surgery twenty years ago, I was expecting the worst. At the time he was given only a fifty–fifty chance of success and ended up with a six-inch incision down his spine, plus eight weeks' rehabilitation. The surgeon gave me a full physical examination, looked at my scans and reassured me that spinal surgery has improved by leaps and bounds in recent years. He said that the operation should be completely successful and that the chance of needing further surgery was only five per cent. He would need to make only a half-inch incision and I would be on my feet within hours. At that point I could hardly walk fifty paces, so even though I was still scared I felt there was no alternative.

Three days later I was operated on. The operation took two hours but as soon as I came round from the anaesthetic I could sense immediately that the pressure on the nerve was gone. I was walking around in the ward just four hours after surgery, had to stay in hospital for only two nights and within a week I was back at work.

Garry says: Disc problems are not as common as musculoskeletal ones but they often require surgery. The centre of a disc is a soft pulp-like material and in extreme cases, like Nick's, the outer edge of the disc ruptures and the pulpy nucleus squirts out, putting pressure on the adjacent nerve root. This is extremely painful and frightening. Sometimes disc problems like this settle down themselves after six to eight weeks – the pulpy nucleus begins to dissolve and therefore the pressure on the nerve disappears.

Unfortunately, Nick's case was more severe and there really was no option apart from surgery. As he discovered, spinal surgery has really advanced and with problems like this is highly successful. The sooner normal movement can be established after surgery the better. Patients are encouraged to get back on their feet as soon as possible. I saw Nick again after surgery and prescribed him some core-muscle-strengthening exercises.

One point of interest in this case history is how the pain became worse at night when Nick was resting. People are taller at the beginning than at the end of the day. This is because discs dehydrate with compression from the upright position. At night-time, when you are lying flat, there is no compression and the disc is able to rehydrate and expand. This actually puts more pressure on the nerve, which is why Nick's pain increased.

FEEL-GOOD TREATMENTS

When you suffer from chronic back pain it is easy to become desperate to find something that is going to give you long-term relief. No one likes relying for too long on painkillers. There are many alternative therapies that people report to be beneficial for alleviating back pain. Most of these therapies are best used as 'feel-good' rather than 'fix-it' treatments.

Choosing one is often a matter of trial and error – some treatments seem to suit some people better than others. Always go to a qualified (preferably referred) practitioner to prescribe a natural remedy for you and beware of anyone who offers a miracle cure. A good practitioner should ask lots of questions about your general health as well as your back problem. Approach the treatment with an open mind and you may be pleasantly surprised.

Homeopathy

Homeopathy is based upon the principle 'like cures like'. The homeopath will spend an hour or more discussing your overall health – emotional and physical – before deciding which remedy is best for you. There are many different remedies that can be used for back pain depending on what your symptoms are. Arnica, for example, is commonly prescribed for bruising and may therefore be a good one to try on the second day of a back injury.

Herbalism

Medicines prepared from plants can help alter the biochemical imbalances that cause pain and stiffness. For example, white willow bark has the same anti-inflammatory properties as aspirin. Herbal medicines can be taken orally, as tablets or as infusions. Dried or fresh herbs may also be added to a hot bath.

Aromatherapy

Essential oils, extracted from plants, are used in aromatherapy for specific and therapeutic effect. The oils are usually diluted in a carrier oil, such as almond oil, and then massaged into the skin. They are rapidly absorbed into the bloodstream and can be very soothing. Alternatively, you can sprinkle a few drops in a bath. As with any of these alternative therapies, apply caution: aromatherapy products can be powerful, just like drugs, so always ask a professional's advice before embarking on treating yourself.

Reflexology

A gentle form of natural healing, reflexology involves massaging the 'reflex' points in both the hands and feet. These reflex points correspond to all glands, organs and parts of the body. Reflexology treats the person as a whole, looking at the causes of the problems rather than just the symptoms. It can be used to relax mind and body, relieve stress, fatigue, aches and pains and aid recovery from surgery. It also helps improve blood circulation and can increase the body's immunity.

Podiatry/chiropody

Some back problems originate from the feet. Corns, calluses or verrucas can cause you to walk strangely, therefore putting your spine out of alignment. There are more joints in the feet than there are in the spine and these are also prone to get stuck, often due to incorrect footwear (see also page 158).

Summary

- It is always wise to see your GP if your back pain lasts longer than three days. He or she will be able to rule out any other possibilities and should be able to refer you to a specialist if necessary.

- If you're prone to back problems, have a regular back check-up.

- The best way to find a practitioner is through personal recommendation. Always ensure that the practitioner is properly qualified.

- MRI is the best diagnostic scan available.

- Less than ten per cent of back problems lead to surgery and if they do the success rate now is high.

CHAPTER 5

Managing pain

Pain is the body's natural response to injury or any disease that damages the tissues. There are two main types of pain, acute and chronic. Most back pain is acute, which means that it comes on suddenly and can feel particularly sharp and intense at first. But don't panic! Acute pain is the body's way of protecting itself from further damage – the muscle fibres surrounding the injured area go into spasm so that it feels too painful for you to move this part of the body.

CHRONIC PAIN

Back pain can also be chronic (long-term) pain. Chronic pain seems to be there for no reason and so psychologically can be particularly hard to deal with. Waking up with back pain day after day is seriously debilitating and wearing. If you suffer from chronic pain, it is easy to find yourself spiralling into depression. Drugs (see page 76) can help control pain but also come with side effects. There are also pain-control clinics to help people cope with both the psychological and physical effects of pain.

Pain is a vicious circle. Studies have shown that mood and personality can affect people's perception of pain. If you are feeling miserable, even the slightest twinge can be perceived as a sharp

CASE HISTORY ⑬

The stoic

Jo, 48, child-care development co-ordinator

The problem
Ignoring pain is good to a degree but when pain persists it must be investigated.

The solution
If pain is increasing after three days, you should most definitely seek the advice of a professional. Your doctor is a good first port of call but sometimes you may need to be referred to a specialist.

I had a very 'old-school' upbringing: my parents taught me to 'deal' with pain by ignoring it. So as a child, if I didn't feel well, I was just packed off to school anyway. I guess this attitude has stayed with me in adulthood and affected the way I first treated myself when I started getting back pains a couple of years ago.

After sitting in a draught I developed a constant pain in my neck, which then spread down across the pit of my left shoulder. It made life very uncomfortable. I couldn't even relax at the end of the day to read a book or watch TV: I'd have to sit on the edge of the settee, bolt upright. Because of my attitude towards pain, I started by trying to just ignore it and hope it would go away. But slowly everything became more of a chore. Even something previously pleasurable like walking the dog became agonizing. The pain was constantly there, although painkillers did take the edge off it for a while. Back pain is such a horrible pain because it is constant irritation, like toothache or earache – totally different from something short and sudden like being kicked in the shins. The relentlessness of it can really get you down. One day I remember driving back from Leeds and the pain was so bad I had to stop as the tears were streaming down my cheeks.

I think people don't always appreciate what it is like to suffer from chronic back pain, probably because it is not visible – it is not as though you have a limp or your arm in a sling. I found it hard to make people realize that I did need to rest for a while. I took two days off from work last week and that, combined with the weekend, did make me feel so much better. Just because you are not crying out in agony, it doesn't mean you are not in pain.

My problem was in the top of the neck, even though most of the pain was underneath the neck and across the top of the shoulder. By leaving it so long it had progressed to what is known as referred pain. If you're in pain, it really is worth getting it sorted out as soon as possible before it gets a chance to set in.

Garry says: When pain is new, it is just another issue to deal with. When pain becomes chronic, it becomes the pivotal point of your life – everything else starts revolving around it. Jo was unlucky enough to experience first-hand what it is like to have to live with ongoing pain. When you suffer from chronic pain, the pain itself can become a lesser problem than the overall effects of the pain on your life. Everyday activities, such as going to work or picking up children, can all be dramatically affected.

Jo is right in saying that many people do not understand just how hard it is to live with back pain. (I've always thought it would be a good idea to have a make-up artist in the clinic painting on some big bruises so that a patient's partner would be more sympathetic!) Most people treat back pain too lightly until they have experienced it themselves – then they know.

pain. If you are happy and distracted by something else, pain is much more bearable.

People with chronic back pain need to be treated with a lot of understanding and tender care. For someone who has spent their whole life running marathons and keeping fit, the idea of not being able to run anymore can be almost worse than the pain itself. It will usually be fine for someone in such a situation to go for a short jog round the block, unless his or her injury or condition is severe. Indeed, the psychological benefit of doing the activity they love most may to a large extent outweigh the potential strain on the back. The key here is making sure that you don't overdo it. Post-injury, the best idea is to do just a little exercise so that if you aggravate the back at all you do so only marginally.

PRESCRIPTION DRUGS

Thanks to modern medicine no one needs to be in severe pain anymore. Most back pain can be controlled with drugs – often a cocktail of anti-inflammatories, analgesics (painkillers) and muscle relaxants. One of the plus points of drugs is that they are so convenient: you can pick them up from your local pharmacy. There are plenty of over-the-counter drugs, but if pain is severe they may not be enough to control it. You also need to take care not to take them long-term as they can have an adverse effect on the stomach lining and liver.

Painkillers prescribed by your GP will be much more effective than anything you can buy over the counter. Always follow the dosage that your GP prescribes and when taking aspirin-based drugs make sure you have eaten something or drunk a glass of milk to line the stomach beforehand. Make sure you take the drugs regularly because they will have an accumulative effect. Pain is always much harder to treat if you let it build up too much.

CASE HISTORY ⓮

Painkillers

Tabitha, 35, film producer

The problem

Taking painkillers is not without risk of side effects.

The solution

Never take painkillers on an empty stomach and if you are taking them long-term it may be worth looking at drug-free alternatives such as TENS (see page 79).

When I injured my back earlier in the year, I went to my GP and begged for the strongest painkillers available because I had to work on a shoot the next day. An hour after taking the drugs, I was lying on the floor doubled up with stomach pain. My husband had to call out an emergency doctor. Upon examination, the doctor said he thought I had inflamed my stomach lining by taking the painkillers. I ended up with three duodenal ulcers, which took several months to clear up. I would never take an aspirin-based drug again and would think twice before trying to rush my body back into action when what I clearly needed to do was stay home and rest.

Garry says: Anti-inflammatory drugs have had such bad press and some have even been withdrawn from the market due to side effects. I always prefer patients to be cautious with drug treatment and to rely more on ice packs and rest. I have had to take anti-inflammatories in some acute situations but I would never advise anyone to do so long term and it's very important to keep to dosage instructions.

Medications mainly address symptoms but it is more important to understand why these symptoms are present in the first place.

Osteopathy is very efficient in isolating the exact structures involved in the pain syndromes. With positive diagnosis, accurate and specific treatment can be applied and pain reduced without relying on drugs. Many people take drugs because they are not aware that there is a viable alternative.

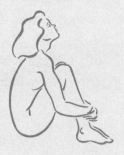

There are also some very effective pain patches available by prescription only that have the advantage of releasing the drugs slowly and continuously direct into the bloodstream.

Your GP may also prescribe muscle relaxants to reduce muscle spasm, which is important, both in order to relieve pain and to enable further treatment. The best for muscle spasm is diazepam but it is addictive and, like other muscle relaxants, can make you feel very woozy because it relaxes the brain as well as the muscles. These drugs should only be taken under medical guidance.

When using drugs, take care not to be over confident about your progress. You may no longer have the warning signals from pain that would prevent you from injuring yourself further.

TENS

TENS stands for Transcutaneous Electrical Nerve Stimulation and works by stimulating your body's own natural defences against pain, releasing endorphins, which are the body's 'happy hormones'. Electrical impulses are relayed from a portable impulse generator to electrodes placed on the skin in the area of pain. I am a big fan of TENS machines as they are very safe and some people really do gain great pain relief from them. TENS is commonly used in childbirth and in treating people with drug addictions.

One of the benefits of this type of pain control is that it puts you in charge: you can increase or decrease the amount of electrical impulse through a dial on the machine. You will feel a tingling sensation but this should be kept to a level that feels comfortable. (See page 187 for further details of this and other types of back pain products.)

CASE HISTORY ⓯

Constant pain

Abigail, 35, artist

The problem
Being in constant pain can wear you down so that the pain starts feeling even more extreme.

The solution
Do something about it by following the advice in this book and seek out alternatives such as TENS, which are safe to use long term (see page 79).

I've spent years being in constant pain from my back so I really sympathize with anyone who has back problems. The pain gnaws away at you and makes you feel so lethargic and scared to move. It can also really damage your self-confidence. In my case, I felt I could not lift my children and I was nervous about carrying my heavy paintings. Even the smallest things change. Suddenly, sitting on a kitchen chair starts to be uncomfortable. I often can't sit down for an evening meal and find it difficult to fall asleep at night because I can't find a comfortable position. Recently, I took my son to the circus and had to stand all the way through the performance because it was too painful to sit down. My back problems are so deep rooted I doubt they will ever totally go away. I have learnt to live with it and not panic when the pain gets bad.

Garry says: Being in constant pain can take away your confidence – a common problem with anyone who has long-term back problems. Abigail is unlucky to have suffered from back problems since her teenage years. Once back pain has occurred more than once, people understandably get very nervous about it happening all over again. It is most important to find some activity that instils confidence in you again. There is natural caution following an injury but, thank goodness, in time we forget about it and life can return to normal. It is the fear of the unknown that is the scariest factor. I find that sometimes just talking to a patient can reassure them that what they do is in fact achievable, slowly but surely.

CASE HISTORY 16

Stress and back pain

Molly, 35, actress

The problem
Stress is rarely a causative factor for back pain but is most definitely an aggravating one.

The solution
Take up relaxation methods such as yoga or meditation. Sometimes just pampering yourself by soaking in a hot bath surrounded by candles can help.

When I first got back pain, I thought it was like a headache and would go away. It didn't and it has really affected my life. I also have a sneaking suspicion that for me back pain is connected with stress – I notice that whenever I feel low it flares up but when I'm on top of the world I hardly seem to notice any pain. Most people have a weakest part in their body and for me it's definitely my back.

About once a week now I seem to be completely incapacitated with pain. Sometimes it's so bad I have to crawl about on all fours. It's very hard for my daughter, too: I've even had to shout out instructions to her from the sofa on how to make her own supper. The pain normally starts about 2 p.m., just before I go to pick up my daughter from school. By 6 p.m. I can't move and then it doesn't ease off again until the next morning.

I have been for treatment with Garry – I was very nervous at first as I was in such severe pain. Slowly my confidence has grown and I've also discovered ways to help myself. At first I would take painkillers, but they weren't able to touch the pain because it was so intense. Now I try to relax in a hot bath with rosemary oil. I follow this with a freezing cold pack on my back. That gives me enough respite to walk about for a bit. It's been a long haul over the last few months but slowly I feel I'm beginning to see the light at the end of the tunnel again.

Garry says: This was a really severe case of back pain, and stress was definitely aggravating it. When I first saw Molly she was in a bad way. I could hardly touch her without her squirming with pain. Acupuncture really helped as it enabled me to ease the spasm and inflammation. Molly looks like a completely different woman now her pain is improving. It has been empowering for her to realize that there are things she can do to treat herself, including working on the causes of her stress. She is managing to have longer periods of relief in between treatments. At the moment she can go a whole week without pain. Once this extends to a fortnight, it will be time to ease back on treatment.

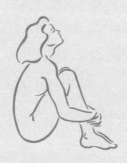

Summary

- Pain is the body's natural response to injury.

- Most back pain is acute, i.e. intense and short term.

- Acute pain is the body's way of protecting itself from further injury.

- Chronic pain appears to be there for no reason and is psychologically hard to deal with.

- Drugs can be useful but do have side effects.

- Learning to manage your own pain is empowering.

CHAPTER 6

Posture

A lot of back pain is simply due to poor posture. If you are a back pain sufferer, it is certainly worth working on your posture in the hope of improving your back problem, or at least preventing things getting worse.

It is well worth trying to encourage good postural habits in children from an early age as bad habits are hard to change.

POSTURE TEST

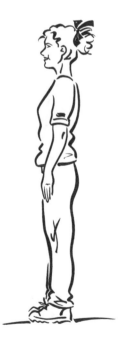

You can check your posture by standing in bare feet with your back to the wall. Slowly press your body back to touch the wall. If you have good posture, only your hair, shoulder blades and bottom should touch the wall. You should be able to place one hand between the wall and your lower back. If you can place a whole fist between your lower back and the wall, or your shoulders touch the wall before your bottom, your pelvis is too far forward and you need to practise the pelvic tilt (see page 107). If you feel one side of your body touch the wall before the other, you are lopsided and need to work on levelling your body out with side bends (see chapter 7 pages 104, 113 and 118) and rotations (pages 105 and 119). If your entire body is in contact with the wall, your posture is too rigid. This can lead to fatigue and laboured breathing. It also produces a lot of tension in the neck, which can cause pain elsewhere in the spine. You need to soften out so that there is a gap between your lower back and the wall.

THE SHAPE OF YOUR SPINE

Not many people have a perfectly aligned spine and there are many degrees of variation. It is important to recognize and correct a crooked spine as this can stretch or compress nerves and other spinal structures. Although you can't change the shape of the spine you were born with, improved posture and regular stretching exercises can help rebalance the situation.

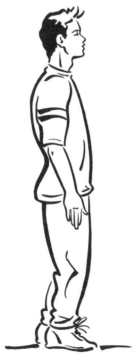

Lordotic spine

Often called a 'sway back', this type of spine hollows out in the lower back. A lordotic spine is common in overweight people (or pregnant women) because the weight around the abdomen will pull them forwards.

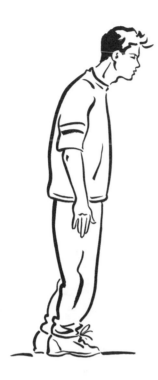

Kyphotic back

This is an exaggerated thoracic curve that results in a hunched back. A kyphotic back can generally be corrected with stretching and postural exercises. A dowager's hump can be caused by the weight of the head and weak muscles where the neck joins the thoracic column. This is often just a symptom of the ageing process.

Scoliosis

This is curvature of the spine: instead of being straight, the spine bends sideways in an 's' shape. Mild cases of scoliosis are very common and can be helped by doing stretching exercises to straighten the spine. As with a kyphotic back, extreme cases may require metal rods to be inserted on either side of the spine to keep it straight and stable and so prevent nerve and other soft-tissue compression.

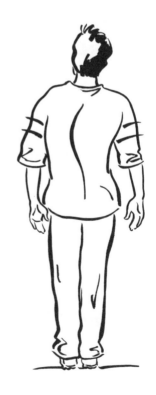

A twisted spine

Pam, 53, teacher

The problem
This may be genetic or caused by carrying a heavy bag over one shoulder, for example.

The solution
If your spine is very twisted you may need to see a practitioner to help counteract the back strain caused by this. Postural methods such as the Alexander technique, pilates and yoga can also be very helpful.

A few weeks ago I was beside myself with worry as I suddenly had this sharp pain in the side of my breast. Fearing the worst, I rushed to my GP, who, much to my surprise and relief, said it was nothing to do with my breast at all – he thought it was musculoskeletal and advised me to see an osteopath. I also had a progressive achy feeling in my right hip referring into my upper thigh.

Garry immediately confirmed that my whole body was slightly crooked. My back, pelvis and knees were all out of alignment. I felt quite a lot of relief after the first treatment, although I found the acupuncture and osteopathy very draining.

The pain is now gone, but we are trying to retrain my body into good alignment. I think that my poor posture has built up over years or even decades. There are not many people who have perfect posture and the older you are the more bad postural habits can build up and cause problems. I now make an effort to stand up straight and not to stick my bottom out. I also try to keep my pelvis slightly further forward. It is all very subtle but it seems to be doing the trick.

I just wish I had known about the effects of poor posture before I started developing back problems from it.

Garry says: A twist in Pam's lower back resulted in her spine bending slightly to the right and put her whole spine out of alignment. This caused an impingement on an intercostal nerve (in the rib cage), which referred through the breast area. This was obviously very frightening for Pam.

Sometimes people beat themselves up because they have bad posture, but this can be changed only when you are conscious of it. I would recommend that someone like Pam practise Alexander technique exercises (see below) to improve postural awareness.

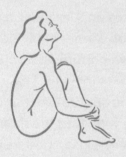

POSTURAL TECHNIQUES

Most people exercise to improve their cardiovascular fitness, lose weight or tone up. Postural exercise is also very important as it can help keep your whole body in optimum health and prevent back pain.

The Alexander technique

Devised by an Australian actor called Frederick Matthias Alexander, who was born in 1869 in Wynyard, Tasmania, the Alexander technique is a system of re-educating the body so that it is correctly aligned. The theory is that it will then be able to function as nature intended. With its strong emphasis on posture, the Alexander technique can be a useful way to both treat and prevent back pain.

When you go to see an Alexander technique practitioner, you will be guided through a series of physical movements, specifically designed for your own posture, that you will then need to practise on a daily basis. Many of these look easy, such as standing up from a chair, but when you start to practise them you will realize how much can go wrong with even the simplest of movements. In the beginning, the correctly aligned posture may feel unnatural or even uncomfortable – you will probably find you have to undo all the bad postural habits that you have picked up over the years – but, with practice, the exercises can make a tremendous difference to the health of your back.

Pilates

A German fitness instructor called Joseph Pilates devised this exercise conditioning method in America in the 1920s. His body alignment exercises proved so effective that the method attracted many professional dancers in New York who were looking for an exercise system for rehabilitation.

CASE HISTORY ⓲

A tall story

Mia, 50, photographer

The problem
Tall people do seem to be particularly susceptible to back pain.

The solution
Avoid slouching and really work on maintaining good posture.

I am nearly six foot tall and think my height has always made me prone to back problems as I have a tendency to slouch. When I first experienced back pain I was in my thirties: I had two young children only a year apart and I was always having to stoop down and pick them both up at the same time. As I have got older, the pain has become more frequent, although variable: sometimes it manifests as a stiff neck; at other times I experience lower back pain.

Most of it, I'm afraid, is self-inflicted: as a photographer I have to lug loads of heavy equipment around and I also spend a lot of time working on the photos digitally on a computer. But I have learnt to do a lot to help myself, too: I started doing pilates, but now find that a combination of yoga and Alexander technique works best for me. The yoga has really helped loosen my lower back, which has a tendency to be really tight, while the Alexander technique has helped me realign myself and makes me sit properly at the computer.

Garry says: Certain body types are more predisposed to back pain. In Mia's case her height has not helped because it has encouraged poor posture. It is good that she has taken up activities to help improve her alignment.

The Alexander technique is a postural technique that is well known in theatrical circles, perhaps because Alexander himself was an actor. He used to notice that around press nights he would lose his voice and one day he noted in a mirror his slouched posture. By changing this position he found that his voice soon came back. The principle of the Alexander technique is to lengthen and widen any area that is being compressed or contracted, which is particularly beneficial for the spine. The Alexander technique teaches you how to use your body properly: for example, there is a big difference between falling back into a sofa or sitting down slowly with control. The latter is obviously less stressful on the body.

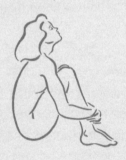

Pilates not only concentrates on stretching but is also designed to strengthen the core muscles (see page 128), which are so vital for protecting the back. Pilates movements are usually performed slowly and with great control and can be practised as floor work as well as on machines. It is an excellent way to learn how your body works and is usually very safe for anyone with back problems.

Yoga

Yoga is a way of life that has been practised for thousands of years. There are many spiritual reasons why people take up yoga, but it also has the benefit of relaxing and improving the body and mind, and is excellent for encouraging good alignment. The Sun Salutations, for example, are a series of flowing postures, designed to be practised on a daily basis, that take the spine through every direction – forwards, backwards, sideways and rotationally. Many people have found that their back problems improve through practising yoga. Always listen your body, however: some people find that yoga actually aggravates the problem. Make sure you tell the teacher before the beginning of class about your back problem. and if anything hurts or makes an existing pain worse, avoid it.

A recent study in Seattle, USA, showed that regular yoga sessions might help combat chronic lower back pain. A team from Seattle's Group Health Cooperative Center for Health Studies assessed 101 adults with back pain. Those who practised seventy-five-minute yoga classes each week made greater progress in getting rid of their back pain than those who did other types of strengthening and stretching classes.

CASE HISTORY ⓵⑨

Keeping warm

Rachel, 24, model

The problem
Over-stretching or making any sudden movement when muscles are cold can lead to injury.

The solution
A warm environment can help prepare muscles for stretching.

My back problems go back to when I was nineteen and hit my head on the ceiling, standing on a stool to hang a painting. I got whiplash from this and my back has been delicate ever since. I practise Ashtanga yoga twice a week and Bikram yoga, too. Bikram yoga, in particular, seems to help because it is practised in a room that is specially heated to 40°C (104°F). Because my muscles are warm, I feel less at risk of injury.

My back problems are very deep rooted and I don't think they will ever be totally sorted. I'm trying to keep my spirits up and make the best of things with my yoga and going for treatment only when and if needed.

Garry says: Yoga has been around for a long time and has great physical merits. Although most people take it up for relaxation reasons, it also provides an excellent stretching routine that moves the back in all directions – forwards, backwards, sideways and rotationally. Abigail feels particularly safe in her Bikram yoga class, which makes sense because muscles are less susceptible to injury when warm.

STANDING

Animals that walk on all fours have the weight of their spine evenly distributed so that it is suspended between the four limbs. In contrast, the upright position of human beings puts a lot of pressure on the spine because gravity is constantly pressing down and reducing disc space, thus impinging on space for the nerves. When you are standing, the weight of the body is concentrated on the lower back, which is why the lumbar 5 (at the base of the spine) is the most commonly aggravated disc.

Try to work on improving your posture whenever you are standing. Pull your stomach muscles in: the more you work these, the stronger they will become, which not only looks good but also helps support your back. Your lower back should be slightly curved but not hollowed out. Keep your shoulders down and your neck long.

Standing for long periods can place the spine under considerable strain. Pelvic tilts are excellent for taking the pressure off the lower spine (see page 107) and elasticated supports (or even a scarf tied round your lower back) can also be helpful. Additional support is temporary and should not be relied on for long periods of time because this could weaken the area. It is important to develop core strength (see page 128) to give you some internal support.

If you have to stand for a long time, slightly broaden your stance, tilt your pelvis forward and keep your knees soft. This will give you a wider base, which will evenly distribute the weight of your upper body rather than concentrating it on your L5 disc. Another good way to relieve pressure when standing is to rest one foot on a raised platform (such as a telephone directory), making sure you change legs frequently. (My guess is that whoever designed those foot rails around the base of bars probably had a bad back and put them there for that reason!)

Inversion and traction

Many people find great relief from inversion, either hanging upside down in anti-gravity boots or in a back swing frame. This can feel very relaxing and allows the vertebrae to pull apart and create more space. Inversion products can be purchased from specialist back shops and sports stores.

Traction is a common technique used in physical therapy. It involves pulling the bones apart slightly to relieve pressure on the spine.

SITTING

Sitting for long periods of time can also be bad for the spine. Try to sit upright as much as possible with your abdominals pulled in for support. Check that both feet are flat on the floor. If you catch yourself slouching, focus on sitting up straight, but don't worry if you occasionally slouch: this is perfectly normal and won't do you any harm providing you balance it by maintaining good posture for most of the day. See Chapter 9: Ergonomics (pages 153–62) for advice on choosing the right chair and the use of wedges and lumbar supports.

Summary

- A lot of back pain can be put down to poor posture.

- A perfectly aligned spine is unusual.

- You can't change the shape of the spine you were born with but postural techniques and stretching can help prevent you developing back pain.

- Standing for long periods puts the back under strain as it compresses the discs.

CHAPTER 7

Exercise

The case for a couch-potato lifestyle can be argued – if you overuse something there really is a chance you'll wear it out faster. And exercise is certainly a double-edged sword when it comes to back pain – it's the last thing that most people want to do when they're in pain or if they're prone to having problems with their back. Nevertheless, people who do no exercise whatsoever and who have hardly any joint pain throughout their lives are the lucky ones and are in a minority. A sedentary lifestyle will do your health no good and you can't expect your spine to function properly if you're not maintaining its mobility.

The two most important types of exercise from the back's point of view are stretching and strength training. Don't panic! This doesn't mean you have to hire a personal trainer or join your local gym. All back exercises can be done at home and will easily slot into your everyday life. Look for opportunities when you can stretch, such as lying in the bath or sitting at your desk at work.

Remember: if you are pregnant, it is always wise to ask your GP's advice before doing any exercise.

STRETCHING

Stretching is one of the most enjoyable types of exercise and is particularly beneficial for your back as it keeps it mobile and reduces most muscular tension. Watch any animal – a cat, for example – and you'll see how stretching is an instinctive part of its day: as soon as it awakes and before any movement it stretches its spine.

Try to incorporate stretches into your everyday life by doing them while you're doing something else, such as watching TV. Aim to stretch every day so it becomes a habit, like brushing your teeth. This will take you only a few minutes and you will be amazed at how quickly your flexibility improves.

Find a time of day to exercise that best suits you. If you like a slow, leisurely start to the day, begin with some gentle stretches as soon as you get out of bed or even in bed – doing a hundred ankle rotations with both feet before you get out of bed each morning is a good way to stimulate circulation through the lower limbs. If you need to slowly unwind at night, do your stretches before you go to bed.

Warming up

It is very important to warm up before doing any exercise as this will make your muscles more pliable and less susceptible to strain and injury. You can do this by walking briskly around the house, or just marching on the spot, and doing some simple mobility exercises, such as circling the hips, gently bending your knees and raising your arms in the air. Try to make all this as fluid as possible – avoid any jerky or sudden movements. A hot bath before stretching is also a good idea.

After warming up, ease gently into a stretch until you feel a tiny bit of tension; this will show that the muscle is starting to stretch.

This tension is caused by what is known as the 'stretch reflex' and is the body's way of protecting itself from injury.

How to stretch

It is important to breathe out as you stretch as this helps the muscle relax. When you try to stretch a muscle, the brain makes the muscle contract in order to prevent it from being over-extended or damaged. The more you try to force the stretch, the stronger the stretch reflex fires and the more tension and even pain you will feel in the muscle. When you reach this initial point of tension, hold the stretch gently until the stretch reflex backs off because it thinks the muscle is out of danger. This takes about six to ten seconds. Then slowly develop the stretch by gently easing into it until you feel the stretch reflex restraining you again. Continue trying to develop the stretch for up to thirty seconds. Remember, for back care, you need to regularly stretch the back in six directions (forwards, backwards, side to side and twisting round to each side).

Floor exercises

If you have a bad back, doing exercises on the floor gives the most support and stability. You can also do some of these in the bath or in bed. These movements are an excellent start to any stretching routine and very soothing for the back. Hold each stretch for up to thirty seconds.

THE HUG

Do this exercise first, to wake up your spine. Lie on your back and lightly hug your knees into your chest. You can start by doing this exercise with one leg at a time and then both together. Now gently rock from side to side. This is a small controlled movement that feels as though you are massaging your spine – your knees should not drop to the floor.

Then, in order to get forward flexion, pull your knees into your chest and hold. You should feel your lower back opening up, which can be good for relieving pain and muscular tension.

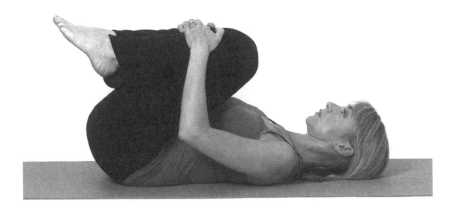

ROCK AND ROLL

Start in the hug position above. Rock forward to an upright seated position and then roll back, aiming to roll your lower back vertebra by vertebra off the floor. Try to build up a smooth flowing motion. This is an excellent self-massage and mobility technique. Don't worry if the movement is only very small at first – you will soon get the hang of it.

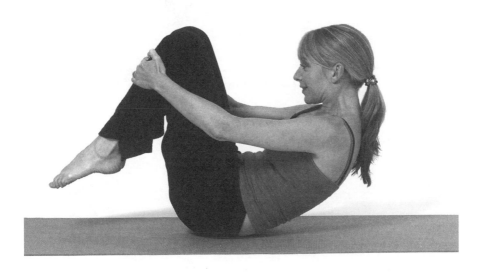

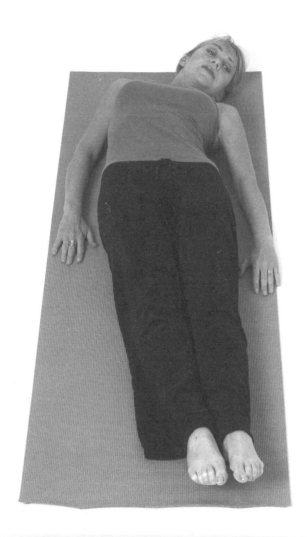

SIDE BEND

Lie on your back, making yourself as long as possible, stomach pulled in. Now turn your body into a banana shape by reaching through the fingertips to the right side, stretching out through your toes in the same direction. Repeat on the other side.

SPINAL TWIST

Lie on your back and bend your knees, keeping your feet flat on the floor. Extend your arms out to the sides. Slowly roll your knees over to one side so that you feel a stretch up the side of the back. At the same time, slowly turn your head in the opposite direction to increase the stretch. Return to the centre and repeat on the other side.

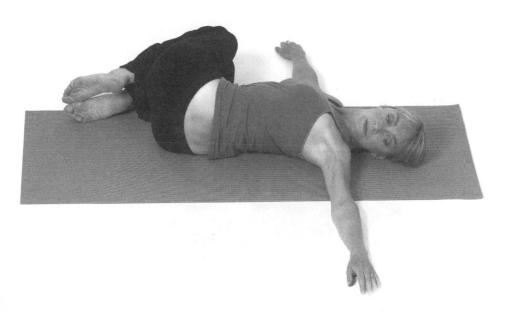

HAMSTRING STRETCH

Most of us have very tight hamstrings, mainly because we sit down so much. Tight hamstrings cause a lot of problems with the lower back so take any opportunity you can to stretch these muscles.

Lie on your back on the floor, with your knees bent and feet on the floor. Raise one leg up and try to straighten it, holding on to whatever part of the leg you can reach in order to pull it gently towards you as far as you can go. Keep your back on the floor and try not to use any other muscles apart from the stretching leg. If your muscles are very tight, you may find this difficult, but persevere – they will become more supple in time. Repeat on the other side.

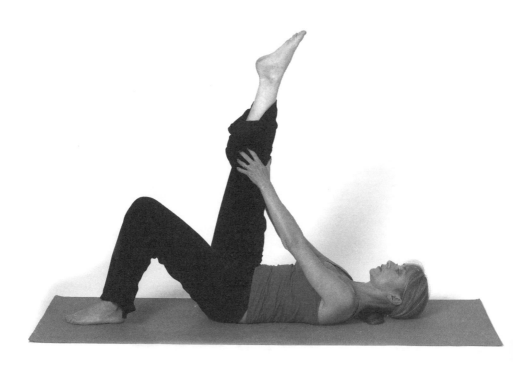

BACK EXTENSION

Turn over onto your stomach. Place your hands, palms down, beside your shoulders, keeping your elbows in to your waist. Use your upper body strength to lift your head and shoulders off the ground. If this seems easy, you can repeat the exercise, this time straightening your arms so you rise up higher. In yoga, this is called the cobra pose. You should not feel the muscles in your lower back contracting. If they are, you are probably coming up too high and are strengthening rather than stretching, which is not the purpose of this exercise.

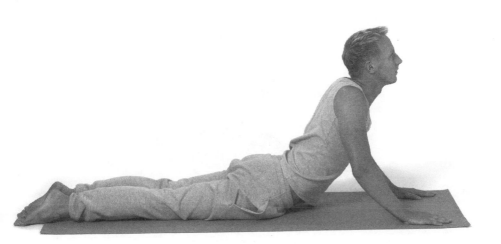

GROIN STRETCH

Sit on the floor with your back straight. Place the soles of your feet together and pull them in towards your body as far as you can without forcing them. Gently push your knees to the floor using your hands and forearms on your knees. Keep your stomach pulled in and your back straight throughout.

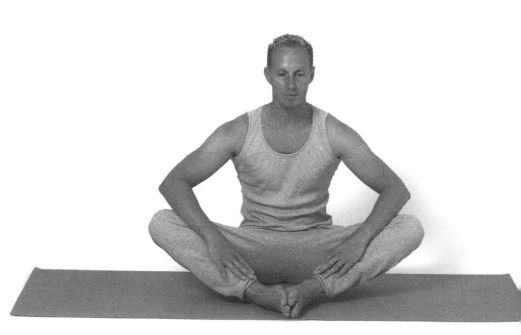

PELVIC TILT

The pelvic tilt is a simple but very soothing exercise to do when your back is hurting. It's also a good way to find your core (see page 128), so practise this exercise as often as you can. The easiest way to learn a pelvic tilt is lying down. Once you get the hang of it, you can also practise it standing against a wall.

Lie on your back with your feet flat on the floor, knees bent. Relax one arm by your side and place the other hand under the small of your back so that you can feel the gap between your hand and the floor. Now press the small of your back into the floor and your hand by tightening your abdominal muscles and drawing your pubic bone upwards. Hold for ten seconds and repeat six times. Practise this exercise regularly until you can do the movement easily.

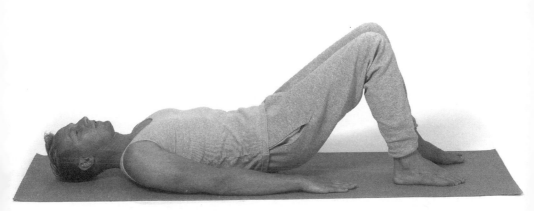

THE BRIDGE

Lie on your back with your knees bent, feet hip width apart. Place your arms down by your sides, palms down. Slowly and carefully curl your tailbone off the floor, pulling your abdominals in as you do so. Lower and lengthen your spine back onto the floor. Repeat five times, lifting a tiny bit more of your spine off the floor each time until you've lifted your whole back off the floor. Think of it as a wheeling and lengthening exercise. Each time you lower your spine back down, focus on the individual vertebrae so that you place each part of the spine down in sequence – back of the ribs, waist, lower back and finally tailbone. Be careful to control the speed and not to arch your back.

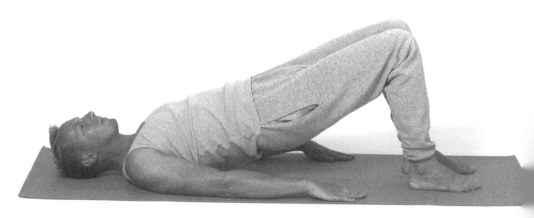

EXERCISES FROM STANDING

The following stretches will take you through all six required directions in the standing position. It is best to start off with forward flexion, which will stretch the joints in the lower back, followed by side bending and rotation. A lot of injuries to the lower back happen when tissues are compressed so leave the back extension (see page 113) until the end because this does compress the tissues and is best performed when the back has already been mobilized with the other stretches. At the end of these standing stretches, repeat the forward flexion to stretch out any tissue that is still compressed. Hold each of these stretches for up to thirty seconds.

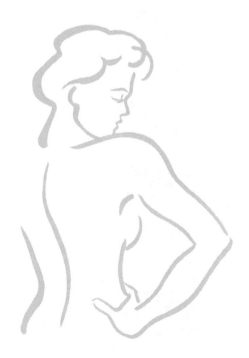

FORWARD FLEXION

Stand with your feet hip-width apart, stomach pulled in, spine long. Reach up to the ceiling with both hands without arching your back, then slowly bend forwards and let your arms reach down towards the floor, keeping your stomach pulled in. Don't worry if you can't touch the floor, just let your head and arms hang. If you have very tight hamstrings you may find it difficult to bend forwards with your legs straight, in which case you can bend your knees.

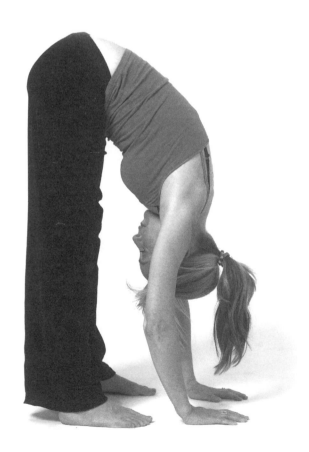

SIDE BENDS

Stand with your feet hip-width apart. Place your right hand on your right thigh. Pull your stomach in as you take your left arm up and over towards your right side. Imagine there is a sheet of glass in front of and behind you to keep you well aligned – your hips should remain forwards and level throughout. Repeat on the other side.

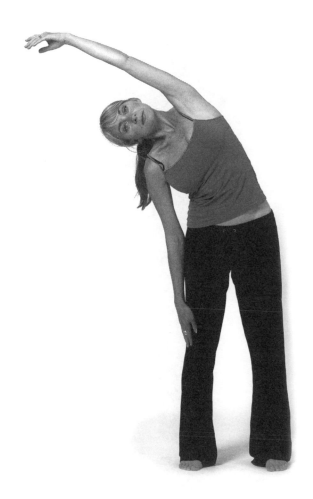

THE TWIST

Stand with your arms crossed in front, hands clasping opposite forearms. Keeping your hips facing forwards, slowly twist round to the left, using your arms for leverage. Return to the centre and repeat on the other side.

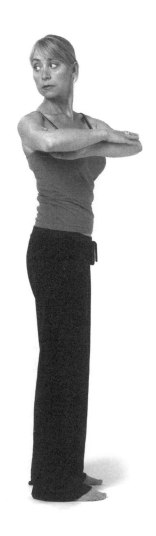

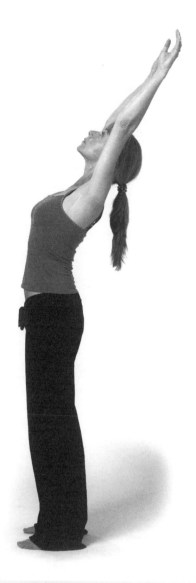

BACK EXTENSION

Stand as above. This time, stretch your arms up above your head, then take them back behind you so that you are hyper-extending your back. Keep your stomach muscles pulled in for support. Be careful that you don't extend too far back.

EXERCISES USING A CHAIR

A chair is a useful tool for stretching. These stretches may feel easier than the standing ones because you will not be restricted by tight hamstrings. The same six-direction principle applies. Hold each stretch for up to thirty seconds. Finish these exercises by repeating the forward flexion (see below).

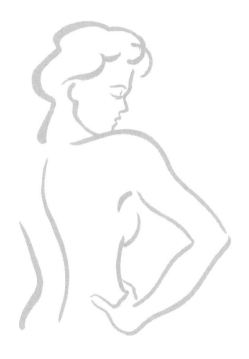

FORWARD FLEXION

Sit tall with your stomach pulled in. Reach up with both arms, taking care not to arch your back. Angle your torso forwards so that you rest your chest on your thighs, allowing your head and arms to hang loose.

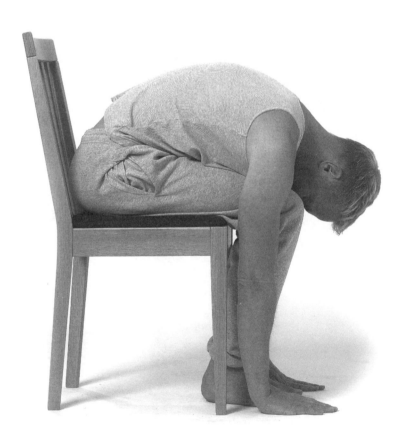

SIDE BENDS

As in the standing exercise, rest your left hand on your left thigh or by your side as you take your right arm up and over to the right. Repeat on the other side.

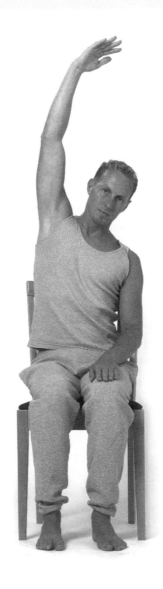

THE TWIST

Twist your torso round to the right using the back of the chair for leverage. Keep your hips facing forwards and your abdominals pulled in. Repeat the stretch in the opposite direction.

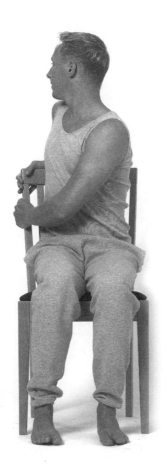

BACK EXTENSION

As you take your arms up, gently extend your neck and upper back backwards just as far as feels comfortable. Keep your stomach muscles pulled in.

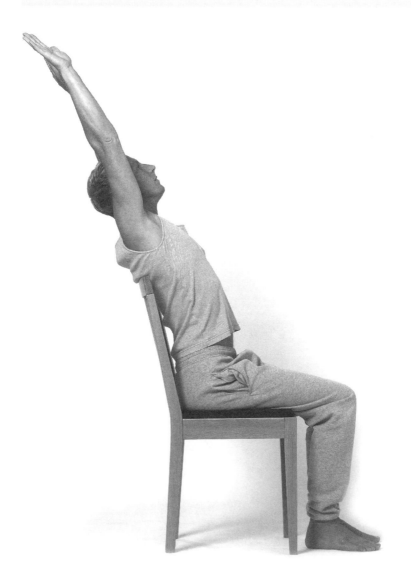

UPPER BODY STRETCHES

The stretches below are excellent for alleviating tension in the neck, shoulders and upper back – ideal for anyone who spends a lot of time at their desk or uses a computer or laptop. They can be done sitting, standing or kneeling. Take care not to arch your lower back. Start by releasing tension in the shoulders by doing some shoulder rolls in both directions. Hold each stretch for up to thirty seconds.

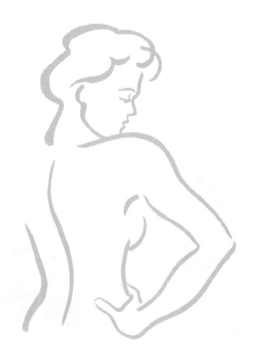

SKY PULLS

Stretch your arms up above you, with your fingers clasped and the palms of your hands facing the ceiling. Keep your stomach pulled in and don't arch your back.

You can then take the stretch out to the sides for a side stretch. Repeat this on both sides.

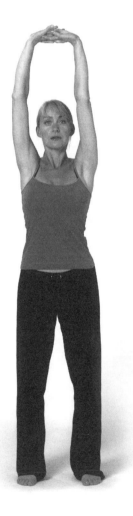
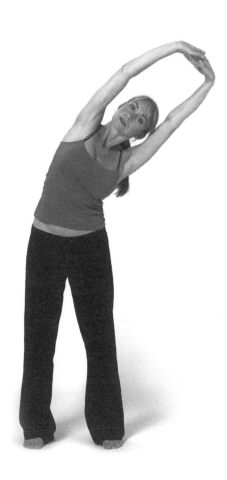

SHOULDERS

Hold your right upper arm with your left hand and pull the right arm over across your chest so that you feel a stretch in the right shoulder. Repeat on the other side.

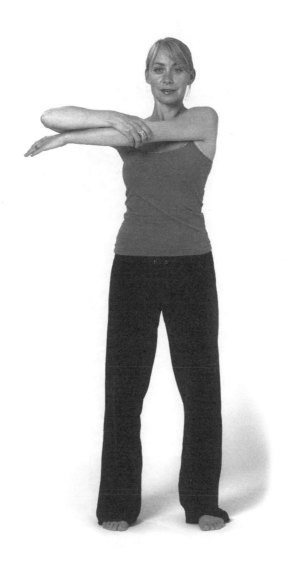

UPPER BACK PULL

Clasp your hands and stretch your arms out in front of you, dipping your head into your chest so that you feel a stretch in the triangle area at the top of the back (the trapezius).

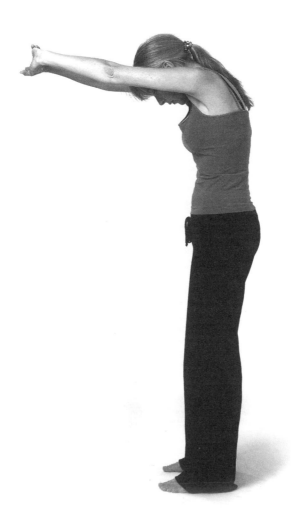

HANDS BEHIND BACK

Stand with both arms straight out behind you. Interlock your fingers behind your back and lift your arms out away from your body. Lift your arms as high as you can, squeezing the shoulder blades together.

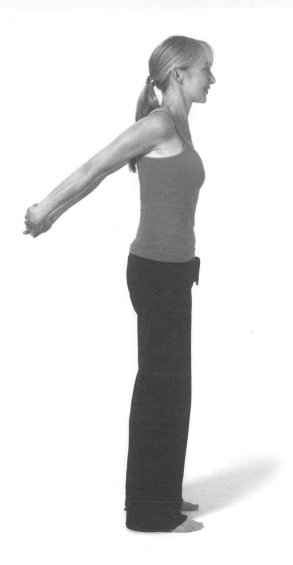

NECK TO THE SIDE

The neck is a very delicate structure so always be particularly careful with any neck exercises. Keep the movements small and never push yourself to the limit.

Keeping your shoulders down, gently drop your head to the right until you feel a stretch down the left side of the neck. You can use your right hand to very gently assist this movement if you wish. Repeat on the other side.

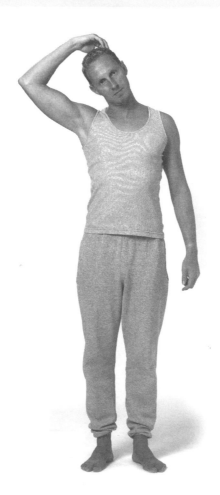

NECK DROP

Gently drop your head down towards your chest to feel a mild stretch down the back of your neck. You can increase the intensity of this stretch by clasping your hands behind your neck to very gently assist the movement if you wish.

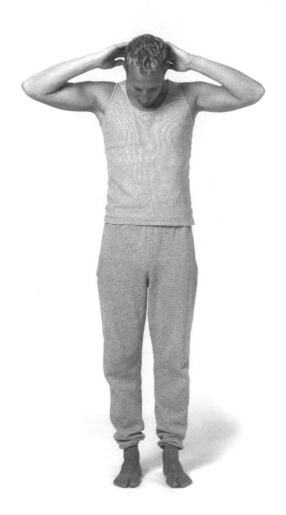

NECK TURN

Keeping your upper body still, turn to look over your shoulder. Repeat on the other side.

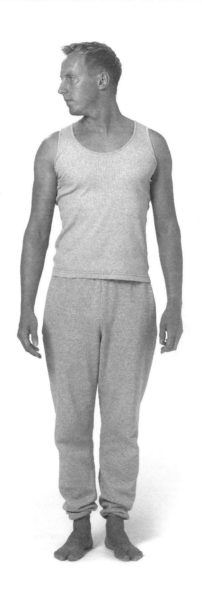

NECK ROLLS

Drop your head to the right and then slowly roll your head forwards to end up on the left side. Repeat in the opposite direction.

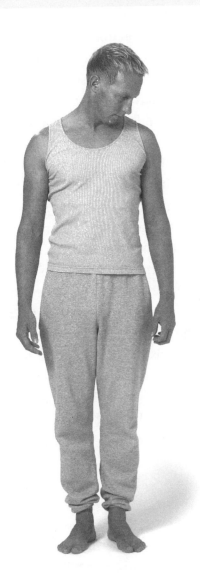

GETTING TO THE CORE

Your 'core' is a 'girdle' of muscles in the centre of the body that plays a vital part in stabilizing and preventing injury to the back. Imagine taking a tin from the top shelf in the supermarket. It's easy to assume that the muscles you'd be using to do this would be the ones in your hand, arm or shoulder. But actually the ones you'd need to use first are your deep postural (core) muscles because these are what would prevent you from falling over as you reach up.

The 'core' refers to all the muscles that lie deep within the abs and back and are attached to the spine or pelvis. They include the pelvic floor, the stomach (transversus abdominis) and a muscle deep in the back (multifidus). You need a strong core to keep your body stable and balanced during any movement, whether you are running, lifting weights or picking up your toddler. Indeed, in order to avoid injury and back pain you need to learn to involve your core in every movement, both when exercising and in everyday activities, such as sitting at your desk. Sitting slumped at a desk all day weakens these muscles by overstretching them.

The transverse abdominal muscles are located deep inside the abdomen and are very important from a postural point of view. The easiest way to exercise these muscles is to simply suck your tummy in as though you are trying to create an inch or two of extra space within your waistband. Hold for a few seconds and then slowly release. Make sure you keep breathing as you brace. Once you get used to retracting your abdominal muscles in this way you can start to incorporate this into other exercises, so that you suck in before even starting a curl-up, for example.

BALANCE WORK

Adding an element of balance to your workouts will naturally engage your core and will improve your proprioception (balance skills), which can both help prevent injury and aid rehabilitation. As well as being important in a rehabilitation programme, balance training is also vital for the elderly in order to prevent falls.

You will need to learn to balance first on a stable surface – just standing on one leg will be challenging enough for some people to start with. As your balance improves, you may want to try some of the various pieces of equipment – wobble/balance boards, balls, decks and foam rollers – that are available to challenge yourself further. (The same muscles would be at work if you were standing in a dinghy with the waves rocking you back and forth.)

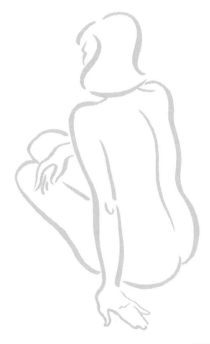

STRENGTHENING EXERCISES

Strength work is best performed every other day as your muscles need a day in between to rest and repair themselves, which is all part of the strength-building process. Strong muscles will help protect your back from injury. Ideally, you should follow a general strength-training programme, targeting all major muscle groups.

Most strength training can be done at home using your own body weight for resistance. If you want to use weights, you can start with everyday objects, such as bottles of water or tins of food. Resistance bands are also an economical alternative to weight sets.

In order to strengthen your back, strength-building exercises will need to target both your back and your abdominals. The abdominals are the opposing muscle group to the erector spinae (back muscles). If these are not in balance, pain and injury can result. Build up the number of repetitions slowly: strength training is all about progression. Don't worry if you can do only one repetition to start with – in a couple of months you will be doing twenty.

The elderly should concentrate on adding repetitions rather than weight. Always prepare your muscles by stretching the muscles you intend to strengthen and don't rush the movements – the slower you do them, the more impact they will have.

Abdominals

Unless you consciously exercise them, your abdominal muscles may be very weak and will not offer any support to your back. Providing you exercise them in the right way, the abdominals respond very quickly to training, and will help protect your back. The following are some tips for exercising these important muscles.

BACK STRENGTH TEST

Lie on your stomach with your arms extended down by your sides. Raise your head and breastbone off the floor and hold the extension for ten seconds. Slowly return to the floor and rest for five seconds. If you can do this twenty times you have good muscle tone in the lower back. If you can do only five, aim for six the next time and add one on each session.

Remember: for best results, strength training should be done every other day as this gives the muscles a chance to repair and get stronger. Stop if you experience any pain during these exercises. You may notice some stiffness the next day, which is just a build-up of lactic acid from the exercise. You can continue exercising once these aches go away.

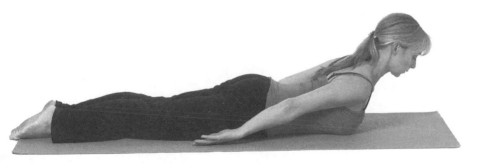

Tips

- Coming up too far in a sit-up is ineffective because you will be working your hip flexors rather than your abdominals. It also puts your lower back under strain. Instead curl up slowly with control.

- Breathe out on exertion so that you flatten your stomach as you curl up.

- Don't worry if you can't come up more than a couple of inches off the floor at first. The important thing is that you feel the tension in your stomach.

- If your stomach muscles start to bunch, you are coming up too far.

- You also strengthen your muscles on the way back down, so make sure you do this slowly and with control – don't just crash back to the floor!

- Sit-up machines can be useful if you get neck ache as they keep your head and neck supported. Otherwise, just cradle your hands gently behind your neck and let your stomach muscles do the work.

CLASSIC CURL-UP

Lie on the floor with your knees bent, feet flat on floor and your hands on your thighs. Slowly raise your head off the floor and curl the top of your spine off the floor. Pause, then slowly curl back down. Pause without resting on the floor in between repetitions. Aim to repeat the exercise twelve times.

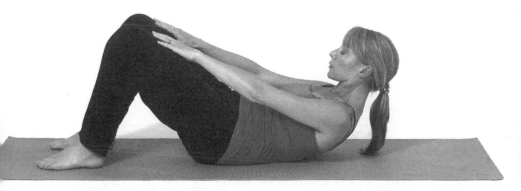

ADD A TWIST

Start as in classic curl-up. Gently clasp your hands behind your head. This time, as you come up, rotate your shoulder so that one elbow moves towards the opposite knee. You should feel the tension in the side of your stomach muscles (obliques). Repeat twelve times on one side and then the same again on the other.

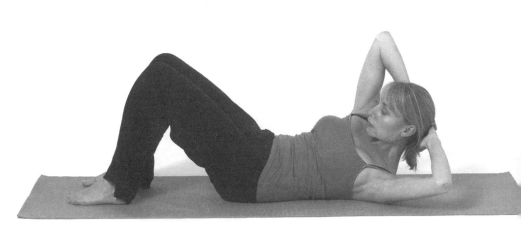

REVERSE CURL

Lie on the floor, bending your knees and raising your feet in the air. This time you are initiating the curl from the other end of your spine, slowly curling your bottom and lower back off the floor. Don't swing the legs – they should remain still – or this will stop you using your stomach muscles. Build up to twelve repetitions.

The reverse curl is a very subtle movement that takes practice. You may find this exercise hard at first, but once you get the hang of it, you can try curling up from both ends of the spine simultaneously (i.e. curling up your head, neck and shoulders at the same time as your lower back and bottom).

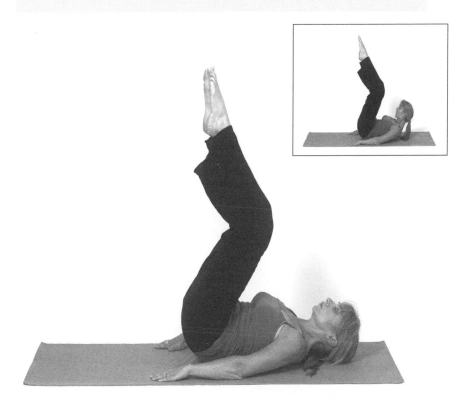

Summary

- The two most important types of exercise for the back are stretching and strength training.

- Take every opportunity to stretch, such as lying in the bath or sitting at your desk at work.

- Aim to stretch every day so it becomes a habit, like brushing your teeth.

- Flexibility can improve very quickly.

- Try to vary how you do your stretches. Practise them standing, sitting and lying down (or, best of all, in a hot Jacuzzi).

- The pelvic tilt is a simple but very soothing exercise to do when your back is hurting.

- Strong core muscles help support a healthy back.

CHAPTER 8

Back pain and sport

One of the first questions a sporty person generally asks when they go for treatment is 'Will I need to give up my sport?' The answer very much depends on what their back problem is, what sport they do and how well they perform it. The physical and mental benefits of sport are huge – for many people it's the only thing that encourages them to keep active. Any good practitioner will be loath to ban anyone from a sport they are passionate about.

Sport can still be a viable option if you suffer from back pain, providing you pay attention to your back and try to improve your technique to minimize any stresses on the spine. It is also worth consulting a professional or instructor in your chosen sport to make sure you are practising it with proper form.

One of the biggest mistakes people make when suffering from back pain is giving up on sport altogether. Although certain back conditions need rest for a few days, most back pain, particularly if it's muscular, will benefit from some activity as this helps relax the muscles and increases blood flow. If you do have a back injury you will need to ascertain exactly what caused it and then look at if and how you can change your training and technique without giving up your favourite sport.

CASE HISTORY ⓴

The need to stay active

Pete, 48, football club chairman

The problem
Inactivity is bad news for the back.

The solution
As you get older it is important to continue exercising as movement stimulates circulation.

I've always played a lot of sport, particularly football. It was when I started having a more office-bound job in my thirties that my back problems really set in. People often shy away from exercising with a bad back, but for me doing sport really did help. I notice my back always feels better when I'm doing regular exercise so I'm sure my cure would be to get hugely fit, but unfortunately I have to spend most of my time working.

Garry says: Pete is very insightful in recognizing that doing lots of sport would probably be his cure. Although it may not be possible to fit a lot of sport into your life, it is true, as Pete points out, that everyone would feel better if they could spend more time being active. I always spend time with patients trying to find a way for them to carry on with their chosen sport or, if that's not possible, helping them to find a suitable alternative.

Warming up

Warming up properly before any sporting activity can help prepare the back for the stresses to come. This warm-up should include some low-intensity exercise (such as walking) and mobility work (such as arm circles) to increase blood circulation to the muscles and ligaments in the back. You should also stretch the lower and upper back (see pages 98–127).

SPORTS AND BACK PAIN

Different sports can place strain on specific parts of the body and, particularly if you have a back problem, it is important to know the effect that your chosen sport can have on your body so that you can reduce the risk of injury or strain. Below are some examples of common sporting activities, the potential stresses they can place on the back and what you can do to avoid these.

Cycling

Potential strains: The stooped posture you adopt when cycling can put a strain on the lower back as well as the upper back (if you cycle with your neck arching back). Cycling across rough terrain also increases jarring and compression to the spine.

How to avoid this: If you are cycling more than just recreationally, choose a bike with higher handlebars so that you can assume a more upright posture, and bigger tyres for more shock absorption, rather than a racing bike. Ask the bike shop to check that the bike fits your frame. Correct cycling technique involves pushing and pulling with the legs; the pulling action is just as important as the pushing.

Golf

Potential strains: The force of a golf swing puts strains on the lumbar spine. Bending over to pick up a golf bag and carrying it adds to the strain on your back. The full golf swing (backswing and follow through) rotates the spine with a lot of force.

How to avoid this: Learn proper technique, including a smooth, rhythmic, well-balanced swing. Use proper lifting technique (see page 166) when picking up a golf bag and balls. You can also buy a special device for your putter that enables you to retrieve the golf ball from the hole without bending over. Choose a golf bag with dual straps and a built-in stand.

Running

Potential strains: Jarring to the lumbar spine. Strain in the upper back and neck can be caused by a poor posture and a hunched position.

How to avoid this: Invest in a good pair of running shoes from a specialist shop, where they will be able to advise you on the most suitable pair for your gait. Make sure you run with a heel-to-toe action, through the whole of the foot. Reduce impact by running on grass or a treadmill instead of on pavements.

Skiing

Potential strains: Carrying skis. Getting on and off lifts and falling when skiing at speed can jar or twist the spine.

How to avoid this: Make sure you are fit before you go. Warm up on an easy run at the beginning of the day. Avoid that last run of the day if you are tired as this is when accidents are most likely to happen.

Surfing/Snowboarding/Skateboarding

Potential strains: All these sports involve standing sideways on and twisting the spine to a degree. Add the impact of falling to this twisted position and injuries are likely to follow. Even water can feel like concrete when you fall on it at speed. Surfers have the additional back strain of paddling out with their neck and back hyper-extended, which compresses the lower back structures.

How to avoid this: Core training is key to help stabilize your torso and improve balance. You can actually buy mini surfboards that you practise on like an instability board – excellent for balance and core strength and very specific to the sport. While sitting at the back waiting for the wave, you can gently bend forward to open up the joints that were compressed while paddling out.

Swimming

Potential strains: Although swimming is non weight-bearing and so potentially kind and gentle to your back, it can still put your upper spine (neck) under strain through poor technique.

How to avoid this: Use a swimming cap and goggles and do breaststroke and front crawl with your eyes looking down at the bottom of the pool to take the strain off your neck. The Shaw Method of swimming (www.artofswimming.com) applies the principles of the Alexander technique to swimming and is well worth investigating if you want to learn how to minimize any strain to your back through swimming and to swim in a more enjoyable and fluid way.

Snowboarding accident

Nigel, 40, event producer

The problem
Snow is fun but not forgiving: many back injuries occur on the slopes.

The solution
Make sure you are fit before you go and that you have good medical insurance. Try to warm up and stretch before you head off down the pistes to minimize the possibility of injury.

I've always been really accident-prone and the fact that I do nothing all year round in terms of fitness adds to the problem when it comes to my annual snowboarding holiday. I often end up hurting myself on the first day.

On my last holiday, I broke a finger on the first day but saved the biggest fall for the day before the last day. I was coming down the mountain at the end of the day and looking up at the lift above, trying to decide whether or not I'd go up one last time. Suddenly I caught an edge, flipped through the air and landed on my back at high speed. Snowboarding accidents have a tendency to be violent, ending with rapid contact with the snow. I fell so hard that I winded myself badly and was also conscious of my finger, which was in a cast. I really thought I'd broken my pelvis at first, but I managed to limp back down to the resort.

I spent the last day of the holiday in the spa. When I got back to London, my back felt really crooked. One of my work colleagues recommended Garry so I went to see him. It was a relief to hear that the problem with my back was nothing serious and, amazingly, he managed to sort me out in just one session.

Garry says: Chronic injuries often necessitate more treatments than something that is sudden and recent as in Nigel's case. He was fortunate that his injuries were not too severe. (On my very first experience of snowboarding I broke a rib, so I sympathized with him.) Because of the way in which he had fallen, his pelvis had twisted on impact. One of the principles of osteopathy is to try to understand the movement that caused the injury and then simply to position the person on the treatment table in a way that reverses this movement so that the body is then correctly aligned for manipulation.

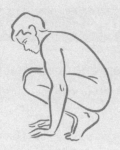

Tennis

Potential strains: Racket sports such as tennis may aggravate back pain as they encourage overuse of one side of the body. Front and backhand shots require a lot of trunk rotation and twisting in the spine. Serving hyper-extends the lower back and can compress lumbar discs.

How to avoid this: Make sure you balance this with some work on the other side. After a game of tennis or squash, for example, swing the racket a few times in your non-playing hand. Do some

Sporting tips

Staying fit and active is one of the best things you can do for your back. Here's how to do it safely.

- In order to get the most out of your sport, you need to build up a good level of cardiovascular fitness. It's useful to keep a track of your heart rate as this shows if you're training hard enough. Your maximum heart rate per minute can be calculated by subtracting your age from 220. For general fitness you should aim to train at sixty to seventy per cent of your maximum heart rate. To boost your performance you should train to up to eighty per cent of your maximum.

- After attaining a good level of general fitness, it's time to get sports specific. Stretch and strengthen the muscles you will be using in your chosen sport. There are many good books on this subject, or it may be worth employing a personal trainer to devise a sports-specific programme for you.

core training (see page 128) to help stabilize your core. Learn about different racket tensions and be fitted accordingly – a more flexible tennis racket requires more trunk rotation than a stiffer one with looser strings. Reduce the amount of arching in the back by using a slice serve rather than a kick serve.

Weight training

Potential strains: Stress is primarily to the lumbar spine from poor lifting technique. Strength training is important for older people

- If you do play sport, you have to expect that you may encounter the occasional mechanical problem. Most of these are usually self-regulating: lay off sport and get some rest and you will generally be able to continue with your sport within a few weeks.

- Following an injury, return to low-impact activity, gradually building up repetition and weight.

- Sometimes a back injury means a change in sporting routine. As you get older, you may need to choose something of lower impact. Don't be afraid to try something new.

- A cross-training approach is much kinder to the back. Try varying your programme so that you walk one day, swim the next and run the day after, for example. This helps avoid over-stressing any one part of the body.

- Buy appropriate footwear as this will reduce the load to the spine and joints.

as it increases their naturally declining body mass, but if they already have some disc degeneration, the back may be even more susceptible to injury from the use of weights.

How to avoid this: Develop good lifting technique (see page 164). Book a couple of one-to-one sessions in the gym to make sure you are performing the exercises correctly. Instead of putting the weights up too high, try to slow down the movement. This will make the exercises feel a lot harder without the added strain of more weight. If you have a bad back, be particularly careful of exercises such as the clean-and-press, dead-lift and squat. When doing chest presses in the gym, always work with a partner who can 'spot' for you and remove the weight if it is too heavy.

If you go to an aerobics or other exercise to music class, be careful that the music does not make you get carried away and lose control of the movements. Always tell a teacher before the start of the class if you have any injuries.

SPORT AS ADDICTION

There are times when it is clear that the chosen sport is really aggravating a back problem. The patient then has to work out whether they are prepared to take the health risks involved. A professional sports person may feel that there is no feasible option but to continue. But anyone who pushes themselves to the maximum in recreational sport, resulting in perpetual injury, is foolish. Some people simply have the physiology to cope with the strains of a chosen sport better than others. If you can keep an open mind there are always alternatives. Sometimes just varying your activities so that you do different sports at different times of the year can really help.

CASE HISTORY ㉒

Living for sport

Joe, 16, schoolboy

The problem

Pushing your body to the limit can lead to injury as well as time away from the activity you are so obsessed with.

The solution

Listen to your body. If you are starting to get twinges of back pain, investigate why and change your training accordingly.

Sport is my life: I play football every day in the week and also at weekends. Out of the football season I keep fit with squash and tennis. All my problems started in a football training session two years ago. I put my foot up to stop a ball and got kicked in the base of the foot. There was a shooting pain up my leg and in the base of my back. I carried on playing for the following couple of weeks but the pain got progressively worse. Most of the time it was just a nagging pain but if I ever tried any sprinting a sharp pain would hit me in my lower back. I was only about five weeks away from the end of the football season and we had a school cup final, which I was determined not to miss. I managed to make it to that match but was in so much pain I had to stop halfway through.

Under my parents' recommendation, I went to see Garry the next day. He treated me six times and then said I couldn't do any sports for four to five months. I was devastated because my whole life revolves around sport. I had to give up the football, squash and tennis and was limited just to swimming. Luckily I do like swimming as well, but I really missed the other sports.

I had been back at football again for only about two months when I hurt myself again. Jumping up for a ball coming over my head, I landed badly and the pain shot up my back. This time it was so bad I could hardly walk. I had to have another four sessions with Garry and once again gave up sport.

I'm now back playing again, but I don't want to tempt fate by saying it is all over…

Garry says: For most children, back problems are caused by a couch-potato lifestyle and also by lugging too many heavy textbooks around in an inappropriately designed bag. In Joe's case, he should have reaped the benefits of doing so much sport but unfortunately the precarious nature of sport means that the chance of injury is only one kick away. Injury can spell an end to a promising sports career.

Lots of young people like Joe think of sport as a golden ticket – think how much money a professional footballer can make! This makes it very difficult psychologically to rest for a while as is necessary after an injury. Sport is important for teenagers as it helps get rid of all that nervous energy and those surging hormones, but Joe paid the price of going back to his training too soon. It was not a good idea to make himself play in the cup final.

The problem with sport nowadays is that we are constantly pushing up against the barriers. Joe is obviously too hooked on his sport to give up but he needs to listen to his body and make sure he warms up and stretches properly before each session. A chilly climate does not help: playing football on a cold, hard pitch is much more dangerous than playing on a sun-drenched beach in Brazil.

CASE HISTORY ㉓

A super-sporty child

Grace, 11, gymnast

The problem
Sports such as gymnastics and ballet can be beautiful to watch but cruel to the back. Sometimes parents push their children too hard, increasing the risk of injury.

The solution
If a child's back shows signs of problems, take some professional advice about whether his or her body can really take the strains of the chosen sport.

'Grace is an excellent gymnast, competing in school competitions all across the country,' says Mary, her mother. 'She absolutely loves the sport but I've always been a bit nervous about encouraging her too much as I don't want her to have problems with her joints in later life. She was training about five hours per week with her school, but if she had joined a local club, as she wanted to do, she would have been training three times that number of hours.

'When she started to get quite a few aches and pains we went to see a specialist, who said she had Osgood Schlatters (inflammation) in both knees. We were told we would have to ice the area frequently but that it was something she would hopefully just grow out of.

'Then a few days before a big competition she suddenly got terrible backache. She had been in an athletics competition the afternoon before and I had noticed that she was sprinting with her shoulders slightly stooped. The next day she had a sharp shooting pain in her upper back and I had to keep her home from school. She was distraught and in floods of tears as the gym competition was the last one before she left her primary school. She was in a team of four girls who had competed together for years and she did not want to let them down. However, I did not see how she would make the competition as she could hardly walk.

'Garry was very gentle with her: he prodded and felt her back while she sat in a chair and explained that there was too big a space between a couple of the vertebrae. He let me feel this myself, which was fascinating. After he had manipulated her I could feel that the space had reduced back to normal. He also gave her some acupuncture to ease the pain, which Grace took great delight in telling all her friends about at school the next day.

'The big question when we left the treatment room was whether she would be able to compete in three days' time. Garry explained that we would have to play it by ear and see how her back felt. Remarkably, she did make it to the competition and their team came back with a medal.'

Garry says: Gymnastics is a very demanding sport and without correct preparation and training it can cause problems to the back and joints. Some children are more genetically suited to this activity. Mary's caution was probably a mother's instinct that had some truth in it.

Osgood Schlatters disease is an inflammation of the front of the tibia (shin bone) below the knee. It is commonly caused by strenuous sporting activity, and usually occurs in boys aged between ten and fourteen. There is no treatment apart from rest and painkillers. Some children who are badly affected are advised to avoid strenuous exercise until over the age of fourteen when the musculoskeletal system has matured.

It was evident from the Osgood Schlatters that Grace was already putting her body under strain. Her upper back problem is not directly related to her knees but it is definitely caused by her sporting activities. Her mother could see from the photo of her approaching the finishing line in the 800-metre race that she was hyper-flexing her neck in her eagerness to win. When I examined her I could feel that where the neck joins the back, the vertebrae was stuck in a forward bending position. A simple manipulative technique realigned her spine and relieved the pressure on her upper body and neck. Again, this would have healed up in time if she had just rested.

Her body was quick to heal, and psychologically it was excellent that she made the competition. I have since heard from Mary that Grace has now given up the gymnastics, which, considering her age and history of injury, seems sensible. Parents must be careful not to push children under the age of fourteen because their musculo-skeletal systems will not have matured fully.

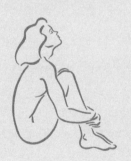

Summary

- You don't need to give up on sport completely, even if you have a back problem.

- Be aware of the strains that can be placed on the body by specific sports.

- Minimize the risk of injury through sport by adopting good posture and technique and always warming up.

- A cross-training approach is kinder to the back, so vary your programme so that you are not doing the same sport each day.

Ergonomics

E rgonomics is all about the fit between the human being and the equipment. As most of us spend more time working than doing anything else, it is important to consider the ergonomics of your working environment, otherwise it can play havoc with your health, with your back being one of the main areas to suffer. Most back pain could be prevented if people took the time and trouble to sort out the ergonomics of their home and working environments.

CHOOSING A CHAIR

If much of your day is spent sitting down, make sure you have a decent chair. Check that it has good lumbar support: you can buy lumbar support cushions, but sometimes a rolled-up towel will suffice. Ideally the chair should be tilted so that the seat slopes gently downwards, ensuring that your knees are lower than your hips, which will bring your back into the correct position. A wedge cushion can be used to the same effect in an existing chair for a much lower cost than purchasing a special chair. Your feet should rest comfortably either on the ground or on a footrest.

Unfortunately, most of us spend far too much time sitting and not enough moving about. Slouching in a chair for hours on end will hurt your back no matter how brilliantly designed it may be. The human spine is not designed for long periods of sitting so make sure you take a ten-minute break every hour and walk around the office or do some standing stretching exercises (see page 109).

SITTING AT A DESK

For comfortable typing, your chair should be at a height that allows your elbows to be about level with the keyboard. An office chair should be able to swivel and should be on castors so that you can easily move round to answer the phone without twisting your spine. Never work with a telephone wedged in between your ear and neck – this is asking for problems in the neck as it puts pressure on all the nerves and tiny muscles.

If you're working at a computer, check that the desk or table is at an appropriate height, too. Try to keep your ears, shoulders and hips in line, with the top of your computer screen just below the height of your eyes.

Electronic desks are available that change height with the press of a button. They are quite pricey but in an office environment they are ideal because they can be adjusted quickly to the height of different workers. The function also enables you to swap positions so that you spend some time working in a standing as well as a seated position.

If you spend a lot of time looking at paperwork, try to avoid hunching over it. Ideally you should have a stand on the desk so that any written matter is at eye level and you don't need to keep looking down or turning round. If your neck starts to feel tense when you're sitting, check that you are not losing correct alignment of the neck by jutting your chin out. This can lead to upper back pain.

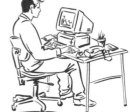

Laptops

Laptops are a major cause of back pain as they encourage people to slump and are usually not used at the correct eye level. If you are using a laptop on a desk, you really should use a separate keyboard and a slanted stand to lift it to the right angle. A laptop is also a very heavy item to carry. It is worth investing in a small trolley case to transport it to prevent strain to your back.

Office working tips

- Maintain good posture – shoulders back, abdominals pulled in and spine long. (The odd slouch is allowed.)

- Check that your feet are flat on the floor or on a footrest.

- Don't cross your legs – this restricts circulation and puts your spine out of alignment.

- Keep your forearms in a horizontal position and wrists supported when using a screen or computer.

- Position the phone on your desk so that it is on the side you answer it to avoid twisting. Avoid crooking the phone in between your head and neck. If you're on the phone a lot in the day, a headset is a good idea. If you use a mobile, use a hands-free device.

- If you have a sedentary job, try to do something active – go for a brisk walk at lunchtime or go swimming or take a yoga class after work. The more sedentary your job, the more you need to balance this with extra physical activity outside work.

Laptop pain

Jenny, 45, partner in a PR company

The problem
Sitting with poor posture for prolonged periods of time can lead to back pain.

The solution
Buy a laptop stand and a separate keyboard and mouse. Take frequent breaks and stretch regularly.

My back problems all started because of my laptop. For years I had worked on a PC with a footrest and a screen at eye level. Then I set up business on my own with a partner. We were very mobile, working in two different office locations as well as whizzing around to see clients and to exhibitions. I was very proud of myself when I invested in a state-of-the-art laptop. Little did I know what havoc it would play with my back.

My back pain came on very suddenly: I woke up one morning and could hardly move – I could look forward and that was it. We had to work at an exhibition that day so I forced myself to get up and about. I remember standing talking to the press with this fixed smile on my face thinking I was going to die. Previously I had been the most unsympathetic person towards anyone with back pain. I never realized how agonizing it could be – I felt totally wrecked. My pain was on the right-hand side of my neck and shoulder, probably from lugging that laptop everywhere. It also hadn't helped that I was always having to look down at the screen.

After hearing Garry's advice I've now bought a proper laptop stand to bring my laptop to eye level and also a separate keyboard.

This seems to have made a huge difference. I haven't totally recovered yet, but I've managed to start running again and feel that life is getting back to normal.

Ergonomics is so important when it comes to looking after your back. I've looked at everything else in the house too – the way the TV was positioned in our bedroom used to mean I had to turn my neck forty-five degrees to watch it. I've moved it now so it's straight ahead and we've also invested in one of those electronic beds so that I can put the back up to support me when I'm reading or watching TV. All these little things seem to help.

Garry says: When I take someone's history I am not just looking at medical details. I am also interested in finding out if there is anything unusual about their lifestyle or if there is anything new they are doing.

If you use a laptop, you are probably continually changing your working environment. Although Jenny used hers at a desk, it was still at the wrong height, which meant she had to hyper-flex her neck. Laptops are handy for work but not good for your posture and, if you are going to use one regularly, you should invest in a separate keyboard and an ergonomic stand to raise the screen to eye level.

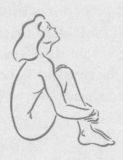

OTHER OCCUPATIONAL HAZARDS

Every occupation has its health hazards. A deskbound job can be one of the worst for back problems, but there are many other jobs in which your back suffers, too. Industrial jobs that involve heavy lifting have a huge incidence of back pain, for example. While not many people will be prepared to change careers to prevent back problems, you should certainly consider the hazards of your chosen profession and try to adapt it as much as possible so as to be kind to your back.

FOOTWEAR AND BAGS

About fourteen per cent of women say that their back pain was brought on by wearing high heels. When you wear high heels, the pressure on the front of the foot causes you to compensate by tilting the pelvis too far forwards. It can put your whole body out of alignment, increasing the curvature of the lower back and thus the risk of back pain as well as foot, knee and hip problems. Try to keep the use of high heels to a minimum. (In the US, you can take stiletto workout classes, specially designed to teach you how to walk safely in high heels. Part of this class is done in trainers and the rest while wearing your favourite pair of high heels.)

Another common mistake is carrying a heavy bag on one shoulder. Ideally the weight should be distributed between your two shoulders, as is the case with a rucksack. Alternatively, make sure your bag is not too heavy and try to swap shoulders regularly.

Repetitive strain injury

Andrew, 51, arboriculturist

The problem
Repetitive strain injury is usually caused by a combination of poor posture and doing repetitive manual tasks.

The solution
Make sure your muscles are strong and flexible enough for the job in hand. If you start to get symptoms, don't ignore them.

My job has always been very physical – climbing and pruning trees. Although I love it and it's kept me fit, the nature of the work has also caused me a lot of repetitive strain injury and resulted in both back and arm problems. It is very strenuous – you have to free-climb the tree, throw a rope around the top, swing on this rope in a harness and then operate a chain saw at arm's length. Not exactly good for your back! In some ways it is very similar to rock climbing but with the added stress of carrying the chain saw.

In my twenties, I started getting problems with my neck and also my forearms, but I ignored the aches and pains and just worked through them. This type of work pumps you up with adrenaline, which allows you to push yourself too far and get injured. Nearly everyone I know in this industry has some sort of back or arm problem.

I started seeing Garry when I was in my forties and realized I had to do something about the constant pain I was in. I was on heavy painkillers and would wake up in the morning with absolutely no sensation in my hands – they would be totally numb until I had been moving around for a while. My neck was also always seizing up so I felt a physical wreck and was mentally very low.

Garry used manipulation and acupuncture to help release my neck and relieve some of the symptoms in my arms. The repetitive strain injury damage to my arms, however, was so severe that I had to have an operation a few years ago to replace the tendons with nylon chords. This has done the trick but means I cannot climb any more: I now stand on the ground, survey the trees and tell others what to do. There is still a weakness in my neck and back, though. Periodically my neck just freezes down my left side – it seems to come on for no reason, perhaps after I've been swimming or sitting in a draught. I'm sure it is as a result of all the years of abuse from climbing.

Garry says: Andrew's is the classic case of someone ignoring the signals from his body for too long because they were all part of his job and he could not imagine living without it. Cutting down trees is certainly one of the most physically challenging jobs, though sitting at a desk all day can be equally troublesome.

The numbness Andrew was feeling was a clear indication that things had progressed too far. When pins and needles become an everyday symptom, it means that there is now nerve involvement and professional help should be sought. Relieving the tension around Andrew's neck and shoulders seemed to help the pins and needles but the damage to the forearms was evidently so extensive that ultimately surgery had to be performed.

The fact that Andrew still gets back problems is probably down to the natural ageing process as much as his past history, but the problem is helped now that he gets it sorted immediately rather than letting it set in. Regular massage would also be a good way for him to relieve tension in his neck and shoulders.

CASE HISTORY ㉖

Pain at the dentist

Nora, 30, dentist

The problem
Sitting or standing for long periods combined with twisting movements.

The solution
A wobble cushion can be a good prop for people who spend hours sitting. Take frequent breaks and stretch.

My back pain is all down to posture. I use a normal chair at work, which does not offer much support. On a busy day I can be sitting for hours on end. Plus I am always twisting round to reach for instruments. About six months ago I got a horrible pain in my lower back, which didn't go away. By the middle of each day it would be a really sharp pain then dull down to an ache by the end of the day. I couldn't afford to stop working so I just dosed myself up on painkillers.

Eventually I went to see Garry, who treated me once a week. After three or four sessions I was able to stop taking the painkillers and I'm now seeing him just once a fortnight. I've started to be much more aware of my posture and have taken up pilates, which has also really helped as it is strengthening my core.

Garry says: Any job that requires long periods of sitting is a potential back hazard. It might make her patients feel a little nervous but one simple measure that Nora could take is to use a wobble cushion on her chair! This would encourage mobility in the lower spine even while she's in a stationary position. It would also help strengthen the core muscles, as Nora has started doing with pilates. She should take regular breaks to walk around the surgery and try to position her tools at the start of the day so that they are readily accessible.

Summary

- It is important for the health of your back to consider the ergonomics of your working environment.

- While you may not be able to change your profession, you should be aware of the potential strains that it may put on your back and try to find ways to prevent or reduce these.

- The more sedentary your job, the more physical activity you should try to fit into your lifestyle.

- Sit on a good chair with proper lumbar support.

- If you're working at a computer, check that the desk is at an appropriate height.

- Avoid wearing high heels every day.

- Avoid carrying a heavy bag over one shoulder.

CHAPTER 10

Life goes on

One of the worst things for chronic back pain sufferers is not the pain itself but the fact that it affects every area of their lives. When you can no longer pick up your own child, prune the roses or enjoy your sex life it really can feel as though your whole world is falling apart. This chapter is designed to help you get on with life and also avoid injuring yourself further.

LIFTING

One of the most common ways of injuring the back is through poor lifting technique. It doesn't even have to be a heavy object – you can injure yourself by bending down awkwardly to pick up a piece of paper.

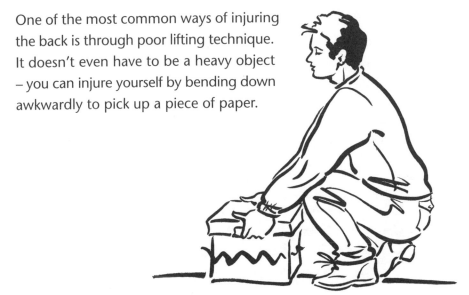

CASE HISTORY ㉗

A heavy load

Natalie, 33, nanny

The problem
Lifting with a poor technique.

The solution
Adopt good lifting technique (see above) and, if the load is particularly heavy, do some stretches beforehand.

Five years ago I was doing a PADI dive course and felt my back start to hurt when I got out of the pool. The next day I picked the baby up at work and suddenly felt my back 'go' as if an elastic band had gone 'twang'. I went to see an osteopath, who did a bit of manipulation on it and then told me to go to bed for the week. It seemed to have cleared up by the end of the week. A few months later I started feeling twinges in my back again. I bent down to pick up the little boy I was looking after and it was sheer agony – I could hardly move. I was embarrassed to ring the woman I work for as I knew she was going out that night – something she doesn't do that often – and I didn't want to let her down. So I soldiered on, although it was a terrible struggle to do anything.

A friend of mine recommended I went to see Garry. I was in so much pain I just jumped in a taxi and went down to his clinic even though I didn't have an appointment. I was lucky that he just happened to have a cancellation and he saw me straightaway. He started with deep tissue massage, which was very painful, but it was wonderful, too, to feel that he had found the injured area and that I wasn't just imagining it all. He also did some acupuncture on me and some of that clicky stuff.

Afterwards I was absolutely stunned: I walked out of the clinic feeling totally normal again. Garry told me to take it easy and not push myself too much, although I felt quite able to do the forty-minute walk home. I was amazed what a dramatic effect the treatment had.

Garry says: Carrying or lifting a heavy weight is a common cause of back pain. It can lead, as in Natalie's case, to a tear in a ligament in the lower back. If you are going to be doing an activity like diving, it is important to always stretch beforehand and to have good muscle tone in the back to make the activity safer and easier.

The second time that Natalie hurt her back is probably not related to the diving incident but due to incorrect lifting technique. When lifting something heavy, such as a child or a bag of shopping, make sure you bend from the knees and not from the back. Keep your back as straight as possible, your head up and the weight as close to your body as possible (see page 166). With a little preparation, many problems can be avoided. It is all common sense really, but you need to do simple things such as making sure the path down which you intend to carry the heavy object is clear.

Treatment is very good at relieving ligament pain like this and I'm pleased that Natalie saw such an instant improvement. Due to the nature of her job, it is very important that she learns to take care when lifting children.

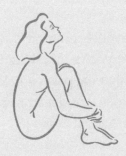

Lifting plan

- Always keep your back straight.

- Allow your quadriceps (thigh muscles) to do the work rather than your back.

- Take a wide, stable stance and squat down, keeping your head up, tummy pulled in and back straight.

- You may feel more stable squatting with one foot slightly in front of the other.

- Grasp the object firmly and pull it in close to your body.

- Keep your head up and push with your legs.

- Stand up in one slow, smooth movement, keeping your abdominals pulled in.

- Maintain close body contact with the object you are lifting.

- When carrying an object to another location, make sure you've checked the route for obstacles first.

DRIVING

Driving is one of the most common ways for backache to start. The simple reason is that you're in a seated position for a long period of time. This means that the pelvis is held in a flexed position, which can stretch the ligaments and lead to pain.

Tips for driving

- Concentrate on good posture at all times. Keep the steering wheel as close to you as possible as this will create less strain on the back when you turn the wheel. A good lumbar support in the seat can help. A neck rest is also a good idea.

- Take care getting in and out of the car, particularly if the car is low to the ground. Slide your bottom in first with your feet on the pavement. Then slowly swivel round to face forward with your hands on the seat for support.

- If you have to get into a car when you're in a lot of pain, you could try placing two plastic bags on the seat to provide a frictionless surface, which will make it easier for you to slide round without the effort of turning your body.

- If you have to put children into the back, it's very useful to have a four-door car. If you can't face parting with your sporty two-door coupé, make sure you climb into the back with the children to adjust their car seats or rear seat belts.

- Never twist round to pick up parcels from the back seat.

- On long journeys, try to take regular breaks when you can get out of the car and do a small stretch routine.

- If you are a chronic back pain sufferer, it is better to drive a car with power steering. If you get pain in one leg through changing gears you may also want to trade in your manual car for an automatic as this sort of pain can lead to back problems. A higher car will be easier to get in and out of.

- After a long car journey go for a long walk. This is not the time to slump in front of the TV.

GARDENING

Gardening is very therapeutic and a good way to stay active, particularly in later years. Unfortunately, it's also a classic way to injure your back because there are so many things to lift and reach for. Make sure you do some simple stretches before you start.

Tips for gardening

- Take care when bending down and picking things up. Remember to keep your back straight, knees bent, head up and the load as close to your body as possible.

- Avoid prolonged bending and stooping by kneeling or squatting instead. A gardener's kneeling pad is useful.

- Use long-handled implements whenever possible to avoid unnecessary reaching or bending.

- When sweeping or hoeing, keep to a forward and backwards action. Unless you have very strong stabilizing muscles, any sweeping motions across the body can put the back at risk.

- When using a lawn mower, use your body weight to help the movement. Look for as light a mower as possible so that you don't have anything too heavy to haul around.

- Watch the wheelbarrow as it's a very unstable design and you may find yourself trying to hold a heavy load that is rocking from side to side. If the wheelbarrow topples over while you are pushing it, you may suffer minor whiplash.

- If your back is playing up, ask a fitter friend or family member to help with the heavy work.

- Take regular breaks from gardening to do some stretches. Stretching outdoors is particularly enjoyable.

LOOKING AFTER SMALL CHILDREN

Although you don't have any choice, looking after babies and small children can be hazardous for the back. But there are ways you can minimize the stress. Much of the advice given above for lifting heavy objects applies here too! Always bend from the knees, keeping the child as close to your body as possible, never twist round when you're in a bent position as this is the easiest way to damage the back, and remember to keep 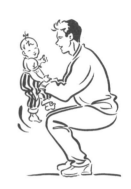 your head up and use your leg power for leverage. If you're tidying up a lot of toys, make sure you kneel or squat rather than stoop.

Carrying infants

Hitching the infant over one hip can cause imbalance and strain in the long term. Make sure you switch sides regularly. Tiny babies are best carried in a sling across the front of your body. Toddlers can be placed in a rucksack holder on your back for long walks and travelling.

Baby care

Look for a cot that has a drop side and is of a reasonable height so that you don't have to bend over it. If necessary, place blocks or telephone directories underneath it to create the right height. Likewise, check that the pram and pushchair are at a comfortable height so that you maintain good posture. When bathing a baby, place the baby bath on a table that is at an appropriate height and don't try to empty out all the water in one go without help.

SLEEPING

Old-fashioned beds tend to be much kinder on the back as they are much higher and safer to get in and out of. Alternatively, you could invest in one of those electronic beds that rise up so that you can read or watch TV comfortably.

Mattresses

Soft mattresses do not support the spine sufficiently, encouraging the body to sag. This can place ligaments, muscles and joints under strain. A recent back pain survey by Italian mattress company Relaxsan found that sixteen per cent of people cite a sagging mattress as the cause of their back pain. A good mattress should be firm and contour its shape around the body, but not be so hard as to be uncomfortable.

Pillows

Pillows should be supportive to the neck. Avoid sleeping with more than one pillow, as this will put your spine out of alignment. If you need extra support under your neck, place a small rolled towel in your pillowcase. Placing this inside the edge of the pillow will help support the curve of your neck. There are also special pillows and mattresses on the market that mould to the shape of your spine.

Sleeping positions

It doesn't matter what position you sleep in so long as it works. When sleep is disrupted it is easy to spiral into depression. If you like to sleep on your back, you may want to slip a pillow under your calves as this will help reduce the lumbar curve. If you prefer to lie on your side, a pillow between your knees will create a more stable base.

Morning stretch

Like a cat or dog, start the day by waking your spine up gently. Lie on your back in the middle of the bed hugging your knees for a few seconds into your chest (see page 100). Now stretch your arms out to the sides. Keeping your knees bent in, slowly lower them to one side so you feel a stretch up the side of the spine (see page 103). Hold for five to ten seconds, then repeat on the other side.

Getting out of bed

Lie on your side at the edge of the bed (1). As you drop your lower limbs onto the floor, push up onto your elbow (2) and then to the upright position using your arm. You may use your other hand to push off the bed for extra leverage. The weight of your legs dropping down will help pull your upper body upright with less strain to your back (3).

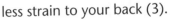

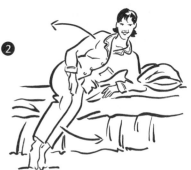

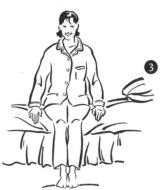

Making the bed

Adopt good posture by squatting down to make the bed. Keep your spine straight, your tummy pulled in and your head up. Avoid twisting. You will find it easier to make the bed, and cause less strain to your back, if you use a fitted sheet and duvet rather than flat sheets and blankets.

SEX

Although having sex is not a good idea in the acute phase of back injury, in many cases gentle lovemaking is actually very beneficial for the back. The gentle rhythmic rolling of the pelvis can be very soothing to back-pain sufferers and this pelvic thrust motion works well as a mobilizing exercise.

Choose the position that feels most comfortable for you. If you both have bad backs, it's best to do it from the side. All fours, with the man entering from behind, is a good position for female back sufferers, but make sure you don't arch your back. The man sitting on a chair with his partner on top will be good for both of you, regardless of who has the back pain.

Sex tips for back-pain sufferers

- Start your lovemaking by massaging each other. This will soothe your back and is wonderful foreplay.

- If you do experience some back pain while making love, don't panic! Just slow down, or stop if the pain is severe.

- Experiment with positions and go with what feels most comfortable.

- If your back is very bad, your partner may have to take the more active role.

Summary

- One of the most common ways to injure your back is through poor lifting, so learn how to do it properly.

- Driving is another common problem, so make sure you sit correctly and use a lumbar support if necessary.

- Be careful when gardening and picking up small children.

- Invest in a good, supportive mattress.

- Sex can be good for mobilizing the pelvis.

CHAPTER 11

Back pain at various stages of life

Your back needs to last a lifetime, so it really is important to look after it. It will be subject to different stresses and strains depending on your lifestyle and age. Your back changes as you age: for example, the discs start to degenerate and lose their springiness, which is why most people are several centimetres shorter at seventy than they were when they were twenty years old. There is nothing you can do about this process but it is useful to understand how the spine ages and what you can do to keep it in optimum health at all stages of your life.

CHILDHOOD

Back pain in children is increasing as their lifestyle becomes more and more sedentary. According to the leading UK charity BackCare, half of all school children suffer from back pain at some time and by the later years of schooling, back problems are as common as they are in the adult population. People who experience back pain as children or teenagers are also more likely to experience back problems as adults.

Tips for preventing back problems in children

- Slouching in front of the TV or playing computer games for hours will not do your child's health any good. Passive pursuits like this should ideally be limited to a maximum of two hours a day.

- Encourage children to strengthen and stretch their muscles through outdoor games.

- Increase the whole family's activity levels by going for Sunday morning walks or playing football in the park together, for example.

- Walk at least part of the way with your child to school. Most children are far too used to being ferried everywhere by car.

- Buy your child a rucksack. Research shows that heavy school bags slung over one shoulder are causing back problems in children because they do not distribute the weight properly and therefore put the spine out of alignment.

- Many school chairs are poorly designed. Talk to your child's teacher about the school's seating if you suspect that this may be causing a problem. One possible solution would be to put foam wedges on the chairs to encourage the correct pelvic alignment.

PREGNANCY

Back pain is very common in pregnancy. There are two main reasons for this. During pregnancy the body produces a hormone called relaxin to help loosen ligaments in the birth canal. This can also have the effect of loosening ligaments throughout the body, including in the back. In addition, the changing body shape puts the spine under additional stress. The enlarging abdomen throws the body off balance and often results in an over-curved lower back (lordosis), while increasing breast size pulls the body forward, intensifying the kyphotic curve of the thoracic spine. All of this can lead to pain and strain in the back.

Tips for reducing back pain in pregnancy

- Try not to gain excess weight. Keep within recommended guidelines, i.e. between 11.3 and 15.9kg (25–35lb).

- Avoid wearing high heels because they will encourage you to arch your back even more.

- Be particularly careful with lifting (see page 166).

- Avoid standing for long periods. If you have to stay stationary for long, rest one foot on a stool, knees bent for support.

- Tying a scarf or wearing a support belt under your bump may help alleviate back pain.

CASE HISTORY ㉘

Treatment in pregnancy

Para, 45, company director

The problem
Pregnancy is a common time for back problems due to weakened ligaments and increasing waistline and breast size.

The solution
Osteopathy is safe for pregnant women. You can also help yourself by maintaining good posture throughout the pregnancy. Massage can also be very effective throughout the pregnancy.

I did not have any back problems until I was pregnant with my first child ten years ago, when I started to have an increasingly painful ache in my lower back and hips. I was a bit nervous about going for treatment at first because of the pregnancy but I was in such discomfort that I went to see Garry when I was four months pregnant. I felt immediate relief when he clicked my back and helped put my pelvis into the proper position again. I went back for treatment every couple of weeks throughout the pregnancy, which helped keep my pelvis in the right place. Ever since having a baby my pelvis has been quite weak so I still go to Garry a few times each year and he has given me some stretches and exercises to keep my pain at bay.

Garry says: Many people worry about having osteopathy while they are pregnant but it is actually very safe to treat people throughout pregnancy. In practice, osteopaths often refrain from treating women at the end of their first trimester (weeks twelve to fourteen), as this is a time when miscarriage is most likely and a patient who miscarried around this time might believe that osteopathy had caused it. In fact, osteopathy techniques employed during pregnancy are very light and both safe and effective.

It was excellent that Para came for treatment throughout her pregnancy as this prevented any major problems. The pelvis is like the base that the spine sits on. If it is slightly twisted, the spine goes out of alignment, which can cause pain and discomfort.

After having a baby, relaxin continues to be circulated around the mother's body until she has finished breastfeeding. There is a theory in osteopathy that a good time to have spinal manipulation is just before you stop breastfeeding as ligaments are then still quite loose, making the body particularly easy to manipulate. For most women, their body will return to normal once the hormones have stabilized.

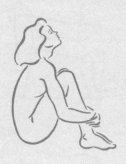

PREGNANCY SOOTHER

This is an excellent mobilization exercise for everyone, but particularly soothing when you are pregnant. Kneel on all fours with your hands and knees about shoulder-width apart (1). Drop your tummy and chest towards the floor while raising your bottom towards the ceiling (2). Extend the neck slightly, then drop your head and arch your back upwards (3).

This exercise also feels great if the pregnant woman has someone place a hand on her sacrum (the bottom of the spine) while she's in the neutral all-fours position. Applying gentle pressure here and making small circular motions will help to mobilize the pelvis.

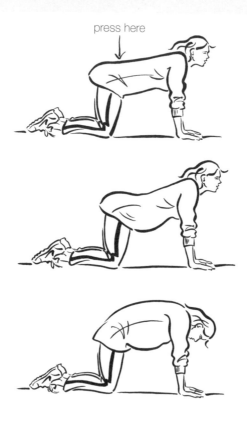

press here

MIDDLE AGE

Women begin to lose bone mass at as early as thirty years old although it may be ten to fifteen years after the menopause that they start getting fractures from osteoporosis (brittle-bone disease). The middle years are therefore vital for keeping up your bone density. Weight-bearing exercise such as power walking and jogging can help. Make sure you get enough vitamin D through sunlight or a daily multivitamin and try to eat a diet rich in calcium.

Middle-aged spread

Loss of muscle mass results in a reduced metabolism for both men and women during their middle years. Putting on too much weight is not good for the back as it throws the body out of alignment. At this stage of life, most people tend to become an apple rather than a pear shape, with the fat gathering round the middle, which places a strain on the lower back.

Diets don't work, which is why the slimming industry is so wealthy – people keep coming back for more. Forget about losing weight instantly. Crash diets result in a decreased metabolic rate – your body simply stores fat as it's scared of being starved. This is why you find that once you start eating normally again you end up even fatter than you were before the diet.

The only way to lose weight is to re-educate your eating patterns. Keep a food diary, recording everything you eat over a period of five days. Instead of eating less, try to substitute some of the more fattening foods – alcohol, cakes, biscuits, pastries, butter, cheese, chocolate, crisps, chips, ready-prepared meals and fried foods – with raw, fresh foods such as vegetables, fruits and nuts. Once your palate adjusts, you'll be surprised what an energy boost you can get from a couple of bananas or a plate of crudités and nuts.

Remember, overweight people are not the only ones to suffer back pain, but excess weight will make you more susceptible.

CASE HISTORY ㉙

Excess weight

John, 46, estate agent

The problem
Carrying excess weight overloads the discs and strains the ligaments.

The solution
Go on a sensible weight-loss programme and introduce some core muscle exercises.

I had to have a major operation on my stomach. Afterwards I felt totally out of alignment, mainly because I was so overweight. I found it hard to stand straight and was always leaning forwards, which inevitably put a lot of strain on my lower back. I tried physiotherapy, which seemed somewhat ineffective, then a solicitor friend of mine recommended me to Garry. I've found the acupuncture he gives me has really helped me cope with the discomfort. He is also encouraging me to work on my posture but it is very hard when you have got into a bad habit to suddenly change and walk upright again. I'm determined to do it, though, as back pain makes me feel so miserable.

Garry says: A lot of John's problems are purely due to the fact that he is very overweight. This not only makes him very unstable on his feet but also puts a massive strain on his back. Although there are many people who are overweight who never have a back problem, and vice versa, it is nevertheless true that excess weight overloads the joints. John is now on a calorie-controlled diet and has reduced his weight considerably, which will help his overall rehabilitation and general mobility.

Tips for healthy weight loss

- Denying yourself certain foods completely doesn't work – you'll just start to crave those foods. Instead, allow yourself a couple of days a week when you can consume some of the less healthy foods or drinks that you really enjoy.

- Increase your intake of water to about two litres (three and half pints) a day. People often confuse hunger with dehydration; once you've had a drink, you may lose that urge to have a snack.

- Eat little and often and avoid bingeing.

- Never go shopping on an empty stomach.

- Concentrate on the food you eat. Avoid doing anything else such as watching TV, talking or reading at the same time or you won't be so aware when you're full.

- Take regular exercise to help you expend more calories and to improve self-esteem.

- If you have arthritis, it is worth seeing a nutritionist who can advise on a special diet to help your condition.

THE ELDERLY

One has to expect wear and tear on the spine, as well as on other parts of the body, with increasing age. As you get older, bones become thinner and more porous. Bony spurs (osteophytes) often grow on the vertebrae, discs start to degenerate and thin and soft tissues lose their flexibility. Osteoporosis (brittle-bone disease) is

CASE HISTORY ㉚

Too old to do what he used to do

Ernie, 62, retired

The problem
Back pain can be triggered by the most insignificant of actions, particularly in the elderly.

The solution
It's important to be adaptable in life. Some of the activities you did in your youth may no longer be suitable.

My back problems started eighteen months ago when I bent down to pick something up from the floor and I felt a tiny stab of pain in my lower back. Over the next few months, the pain did diminish but I still felt there was something wrong so I went to see Garry, who was recommended to me by my daughter-in-law. The pain was always aggravated by bending forwards, which made everyday things like gardening difficult. This would often lead to a pain in the thigh area, too.

I've now had four sessions over six weeks. I no longer get such a reaction when I'm gardening and feel my back is getting stronger again. Garry has given me some exercises, which I make sure I do regularly. It still doesn't feel completely cured, so for my peace of mind I am going to get a medical diagnosis, probably a scan, done soon.

I've had to change my lifestyle – I was a runner for twenty years – now I just power walk and swim, which doesn't seem to annoy my back so much. I do miss the running but there are benefits too – it used to give me exercise-induced asthma, which has gone now. I think you have to be adaptable in life. If you have a back problem when you're older it is often more a case of managing it than finding a complete cure.

Garry says: As Ernie has perceptively commented, as you age, a cure becomes less likely and it becomes more important to manage your back correctly. He has a healthy approach to adapting to the needs of his age.

It is good that Ernie has switched from running to lower impact exercises. Low-impact or non-weight-bearing exercise is preferable in later life, as it does not place as much strain on the joints and surrounding structures as high-impact or weight-bearing activities. Suppleness, strength and balance become the key issues. Exercising in water is ideal as the limbs are supported, enabling you to achieve a greater range of movement with less risk of injury. The resistance of the water will aid in the strengthening of the muscles and so prevent injury on dry land.

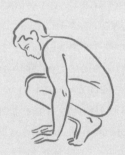

common over the age of fifty, especially in women. Your bones become lighter as you age: by the time you are seventy, your bones are about a third lighter than they were at the age of forty. Muscle mass also declines, which is why it is important to keep exercising.

The elderly should do some weight-bearing exercise, such as walking (full-impact activity such as running is too much for most older frames) and also some strength training to keep up muscle mass. Swimming is a good general exercise that is ideal for fragile bones as it's non-impact. At this time of life, maintaining suppleness and mobility is vital. Daily stretching and mobility routines can make a tremendous difference to wellbeing.

Preventative treatment is recommended: physiotherapy is excellent for ensuring you keep all your joints mobile. An elderly person with back pain can also be treated with physical therapies such as osteopathy but this has to be approached very gently using passive techniques rather than high-velocity thrusts.

When you're young, you can fall over hard and just get up and carry on. When you're old, falling can be the beginning of the end. Unfortunately, we become more unstable as we grow old and more prone to falling. Elderly people need to work hard at maintaining good postural habits and muscle tone. If there is any time in your life that you need to stay active, it's now.

Summary

- Sedentary lifestyles are putting children's health at risk and causing back problems. Limit passive pursuits such as watching TV and playing computer games and ensure that your child gets plenty of exercise.

- Pregnancy puts the back in a more vulnerable state due to an increase in a hormone called relaxin and enlarging abdomen and breast size.

- The middle years are vital for keeping up your bone density: make sure you are doing some weight-bearing exercise and getting enough vitamin D.

- Weight gain, which can become a problem in middle age, puts extra strain on the back.

- It is important to stay active in later life. Focus on maintaining suppleness, strength and balance and avoid weight-bearing exercise. Accept that you may need to make some adjustments to your lifestyle.

Products that might help

There is a huge market for back-pain products. While some of these are pricey gimmicks that really aren't much use at all, there are others that really do have a value. Here is a list of the top ten products to invest in:

1 **Wobble board** The definitive exercise tool that will improve your balance and core stability. It will also help strengthen your lower limbs and so help prevent the chance of back injury.

2 **TENS machine** A non-drug form of pain relief that stimulates the body's own natural painkiller, endorphins.

3 **Lumbar roll** For using in a chair or car seat. It allows the back muscles to relax and be supported while you are in a seated position. There are numerous ones on the market including inflatable ones for travel.

4 **Devil's claw** A herbal remedy that really does have fantastic research behind it to support its traditional usage for relief of muscular aches and pains, particularly back pain.

5 **Massage machine** If you've got no one to do it for you, invest in a hand-held machine. This is ideal for boosting circulation and reducing muscular tension.

6   **Glucosamine** Glucosamine is a naturally occurring amino sugar that is vital to the body's connective tissue. While symptoms are acute take about 1500mg of glucosamine daily, reducing to 500mg daily for maintenance. You can also buy glucosamine in patch form so that it is instantly absorbed into the bloodstream at the site of pain. There are many clinical studies that show the efficacy and safety of taking glucosamine.

7   **Magnets** There have been numerous studies to show how magnets can help with pain relief by increasing blood flow to the painful area. There are various magnetic products on the market that can be useful for back pain sufferers including in-lays for the mattress and pillow, magnets to place on the site of pain and magnetic wands that work by an electronic pulse.

8   **Ice/heat packs** Both ice and heat can help with reducing pain. Wheat bags are useful for heating up in the microwave. You can also buy packs that can be both heated and iced, depending on your symptoms.

9   **Balance ball** Another great rehabilitation tool for anyone with a back problem. This is ideal for practising core stability exercises on. Make sure you buy one that comes with an instructional video, or book a one-to-one session with a personal trainer who will be able to teach you what to do.

10 **Wedge** This will encourage good posture when seated by raising the pelvis slightly higher than the knees. This assists circulation in the legs and encourages the spine's curvature into its natural shape. This product is ideal if you have to spend a lot of time seated at a desk.

Further Information

UK

BackCare (020 8977 5474;
www.backcare.org.uk)
Independent national charity for people
with back pain.

British Acupuncture Council (020
8735 0400; www.acupuncture.org.uk)
UK's main regulatory body for the
practice of traditional acupuncture.

British Chiropractic Association
(0118 950 5950;
www.chiropractic-uk.co.uk) Largest and
longest established association for
chiropractors in the UK.

**Chartered Society of
Physiotherapy** (020 7306 6666;
www.csp.org.uk) Largest and longest-
established association for
physiotherapists in the UK.

General Osteopathic Council
(020 7357 6655; www.osteopathy.org.uk)
Professional body of osteopathy.

Pain Concern UK (01620 822572;
www.painconcern.org.uk) Information
and support for pain sufferers and those
who care for them. Provide free fact-
sheet and leaflets to help you manage
your pain.

**Society of Teachers of the
Alexander Technique**
(0845 230 7828; www.stat.org.uk)

Spinal Injuries Association
(www.spinal.co.uk)
Counselling Helpline 0800 980 0501.

AUSTRALIA

**ABC – Health Matters Library
Fact File**
(www.abc.net.au/health/library/backpain
_ff.htm)
General information about back pain and
the ability to search for recent ABC
reports on developments in back care.

**Australian Acupuncture &
Chinese Medicine Association**
(1300 725 334;
www.acupuncture.org.au) Professional
organisation representing acupuncture
and traditional Chinese medicine
practitioners in Australia. Includes
practitioner search function.

**Australian Natural Therapists
Association** (1800 817 577;
www.anta.com.au) Established in 1955,
this is a professional body of alternative
and complementary medical

practitioners and therapists. Includes a practitioner search function.

Australian Osteopathic Association (1800 467 836;

www.osteopathic.com.au) Founded in 1955, the AOA represents Australian osteopaths in all states. Includes a practitioner search function.

Australian Physiotherapy Association ((03) 9534 9400;

www.apa.advsol.com.au) Peak body representing the interests of Australian physiotherapists and their patients. Includes a search function to help you find a local physio.

Australian Society of Teachers of the Alexander Technique

((03) 9499 7566
http://www.austat.org.au/) Gives further information about techniques and provides search function to find local listed practitioner.

Chiropractors Association of Australia ((02) 4731 8011;

www.chiropractors.asn.au) Professional association for Australian chiropractors.

NEW ZEALAND

Association of New Zealand Teachers of the Alexander Technique (09 846 9727;

www.alexandertechnique.gen.nz)

New Zealand Chiropractors' Association (09 360 2089;

www.chiropractic.org.nz)

New Zealand Pain Society Inc

(info@nzps.org.nz; www.nzps.org.nz) Promotes education, training, research and development in all areas of pain.

Pain Action in New Zealand

(03 3660 716;
homepages.ihug.co.nz/~procter/PAINZ. HTM)

New Zealand Register of Acupuncturists (04 476 4866;

www.acupuncture.org.nz)

New Zealand Society of Physiotherapists Inc (04 8016500;

nzsp.org.nz)

New Zealand Spinal Trust (03 383

6881; www.nzspinaltrust.org.nz) Provides information, education, research, advocacy and support for people who have spinal cord impairment.

Osteopathic Council of New Zealand (04 474 0747;

www.osteopathiccouncil.org.nz) Regulates the osteopathic profession and maintains a public register of osteopaths.

Index